DISCLAIMER

The Hospice and Palliative Nurses Association,
its officers and directors and the authors and
reviewers of this core curriculum make no claims
that buying or studying it will guarantee a passing
score on the CHPLN Certification examination.

INTRODUCTION

Working in many settings, including long-term care, hospitals, and home care and hospice, licensed practical/vocational nurses play a central role in providing care to very sick and/or dying patients and their families. The cornerstone of their practice is the provision of evidence-based physical, emotional, psychosocial and spiritual care in collaboration with the family, RN and other members of the healthcare team. Because of their consistent interaction with the patients and families, LP/VN's are well positioned to observe the physical and psychosocial symptoms that are common to those who are very sick and/or terminal. They also see first hand the existential and spiritual issues with which the patients and their families struggle. They regularly witness and experience the profound, multiple losses and grief that accompany the dying process.

The purpose of the *Core Curriculum for the Licensed Practical/Vocational Hospice and Palliative Nurse* is to recognize the LP/VN's role in palliative and end-of-life care, and to ensure adequate preparation and educational support for their work.

We realized that one of our biggest challenges was to address the diversity among LP/VN's. Practice and expertise differ based on geographic area and clinical setting, as well as the individual's cultural, educational, and experiential background. To help you understand how we incorporated these variations and made decisions about the depth and breadth of information, we want to make explicit the principles that guided the development of the *Core Curriculum*. We believe that:

- Better educational preparation for LP/VN's results in more effective care to dying patients and their families.

- LP/VN's are integral members of the hospice and palliative care team. In order to participate actively in planning and providing quality end-of-life care, they need to possess a thorough knowledge of hospice and palliative care concepts and practices.

- LP/VN's who are educated and involved in the care of dying patients experience greater job satisfaction, which may in turn decrease job turnover that threatens the quality and consistency of end-of-life care.

- LP/VN's do not make decisions about medical therapies; however they are to "demonstrate decision making in the care of patients and families experiencing life-limiting, progressive illness through use of the nursing process to address the physical, emotional, psychosocial, and spiritual needs of the patients and families."[1,p1] In addition, their attitudes towards certain therapies, such as opioids and artificial nutrition, are communicated either directly or indirectly to patients and families. Thus, they need to be aware of the reasons for instituting or withdrawing therapies and to realize that their attitudes influence patients and families. For this reason, the *Core Curriculum for the Licensed Practical/Vocational Hospice and Palliative Nurse* contains information about medical therapies for several symptoms.

- Our goal is to ensure competent, professional end-of-life care. We understand that the knowledge and skill level suggested by some of the content may exceed your scope of practice in some settings. However, we present these materials to set the standard. Our experience as clinicians, educators, and researchers has shown us that many LP/VN's are deeply committed to their work and want to provide a high level of end-of-life care, not merely the minimum. This *Core Curriculum* was developed to reflect this goal.

This review manual is authored by credible experts from the field of hospice and palliative care. It has been reviewed by experts in these fields as well, in addition to education and pharmacy. This *Core Curriculum* is recognized as one of many excellent resources to be used in preparing for professional assessment activities. As you read through the chapters, please remember that you are to "reflect the scope and standards of hospice and palliative care under the direction of a registered nurse"[2,p7] as put forth in the *Statement on the Scope and Standards of Hospice and Palliative Licensed Practical/Vocational Nursing Practice.*

There are thirteen chapters covering 1) Overview of Hospice and Palliative Care, 2) Interdisciplinary Collaboration, 3) Patterns of Disease Progression, 4) Pain, 5) Other Symptoms, 6) Communication, 7) Culture, 8) Spirituality, 9) Pediatrics, 10) Family Caregivers, 11) Loss and Bereavement, 12) Time of Death: Indicators of Imminent Death, and 13) Personal and Professional Development. In the *Study Guide for the Licensed Practical/Vocation Hospice and Palliative Nurse*, questions are provided that correspond with each chapter that helps the student synthesize the information. Answers are provided as well, along with rationales to ensure the correct information is learned. There are also case studies with questions and answer rationales in the *Study Guide*. We hope you will find this manual very useful and best wishes for a successful exam.

The scope of this project necessitates much help thereby warranting many "thank you's." We are very grateful to all of the contributing authors who willingly gave of their time and expertise, as well as the reviewers for their hard work. A special thank you to Judy Lentz, CEO of HPNA and Amy Killmeyer, Assistant Administrator/ Office Manager for their support of this project.

Tami Borneman, RN, MSN, CNS
Dena Jean Sutermaster, RN, MSN, CHPN®

CITED REFERENCES

1. Dahlin C, Lentz J, Sutermaster DJ. *Professional Competencies for the Hospice and Palliative Licensed Practical/Vocational Nurse.* Dubuque, IA: Kendall/Hunt Publishing Company; 2004.

2. Dahlin C, Lentz J, Sutermaster DJ. *Statement of the Scope and Standards of Hospice and Palliative Licensed Practical/Vocational Nursing Practice.* Dubuque, IA: Kendall/Hunt Publishing Company; 2004.

CHAPTER I

AN OVERVIEW OF HOSPICE AND PALLIATIVE CARE

Tami Borneman, RN, MSN, CNS

Adapted from: Volker BG, Watson AC. An overview of hospice and palliative care.
Core Curriculum for the Hospice and Palliative Nurse. 2nd ed. Dubuque, IA: Kendall/Hunt; in press.

I. **History of Hospice and Palliative Care**

A. **Hospice**

1. Concept antedates 475 AD

2. The term "hospes," from which the term hospice is derived, means to be both host and guest; implies an interaction and mutual caring between patient, family and hospice staff

3. Self-sustained communities evolved after 335 AD where ill, weary, homeless and dying persons received care

4. During the early middle ages, words *hospice, hospital* and *hostel* were used interchangeably

5. Also during the middle ages *hospitia,* or traveler's rests provided food, shelter, as well as care for those sick or dying

6. The care and support of the whole person (the soul, mind, spirit) evolved in these early hospices

7. Evolved to care for the sick and incurables in 1800's

8. The word hospice became synonymous with care of the terminally ill late in the 1800's with the founding of Our Lady's Hospice in Dublin by Sister May Aikenhead of the Irish Sisters of Charity, who was a colleague of Florence Nightingale

9. St. Joseph's Hospice established in 1900 in London; Dame Cicely Saunders began refining the ideas and protocols that formed the cornerstone of modern hospice care in the 1950's and 60's

10. Cicely Saunders, MD opened St. Christopher's Hospice in the 1960's in suburban London, marking the beginning of the modern hospice movement

11. Cicely Saunders, MD visited the US in 1963 and spoke to the medical and nursing students, and interested others at Yale University

12. Florence Wald, Dean of Yale School of Nursing, resigned to plan and found the Connecticut Hospice

13. The Palliative Care service at the Royal Victoria Hospital, Montreal, Canada, started by Balfour Mount, MD opened in 1975; first use of the term "palliative care" to refer to a program of care for terminally ill persons and their families; this became the first hospice in North America

14. The Connecticut Hospice incorporated in 1971, began seeing home care patients in 1974, 44 bed inpatient facility opened in 1979; the first hospice in the US

15. 1983 Tax Equity Fiscal Responsibility Act created the Medicare Hospice Benefit; defines hospice care in the US

B.   Palliative Care

1. David Tasma, a Polish Jew who died of cancer in a London hospital in 1948—left Cicely Saunders a small legacy, saying, "I want to be a window in your home."

2. She acknowledges her interaction with him as the beginning of her work with thousands of dying patients, from which she established science of palliative medicine

   a) Attends to the whole person

   b) Is limited to those who have progressive predictable disease

   c) Uses scientific rigor in developing treatment for pain and symptoms[1]

3. Contrasting views exist about the evolution of palliative care

   a) Hospice and palliative care are often seen as synonymous, e.g., in England and Canada, hospice is also called palliative care[2]

   b) Hospice is thought to be a subset of palliative care[3]

   c) Palliative care found its roots in hospice[4]

   d) Hospice includes the elements of palliative care, but not all palliative care includes all the elements of hospice care[5]

II.   Development of Modern Hospice and Palliative Care Movements

A.   Hospice Landmark Events

1. Development of current concepts of palliative care are, in large part, through the work of Dame Cicely Saunders at St. Christopher's Hospice in London, including the use of scheduled oral opioids for pain management

2. Elisabeth Kübler-Ross's work in the 1960's demystified death and dying and opened the debate on care of the dying for healthcare professionals and the lay public; *On Death and Dying* was published in 1969

3. Increased knowledge and research regarding grief, loss, and bereavement

4. General dissatisfaction (among the public and some factions of the healthcare system) about how dying persons and their families are treated in the US healthcare system which generally emphasizes technological intervention and over treatment to prevent death

5. Development of the holistic nursing practice model

6. Issues related to cost of care versus quality of life

7. Physician assisted suicide movement and the 1995 results of the SUPPORT study, showing high incidence of uncontrolled pain (from 74% to 95%) in very ill and dying adults in spite of planned interventions from nurses to encourage physicians to attend to pain control[6]

8. The "natural death" consumer movement similar to the natural childbirth movement

9. Publication by the National Hospice Organization (NHO) of *A Pathway for Patients and Families Facing Terminal Illness* (1997)

10. Development by the National Hospice and Palliative Care Organization (NHPCO) of *Hospice Standards of Practice* (2001)

B.   Palliative Care

1. Major factors have influenced the recent development of palliative care programs in the United States

   a) Consumer demand

      i. Aging of the population

      ii. Growing public interest in assisted suicide and euthanasia

      iii. Growing gap between what people with life-threatening illness desire and what they experience from healthcare systems and providers

      iv. Supreme Court's ruling on the right to die and its affirmation of right to care at the end of life

   b) Acknowledgment by medical community that care of dying is poor

      i. SUPPORT Study results[6]

      ii. 1997 Institute of Medicine's report on End-of-life Care[7]

      iii. Development of WHO Standards for Cancer Pain Relief (1996)[8]

      iv. 1990 WHO guidelines on Cancer Pain Relief and Palliative Care[8]

      v. AHCPR Cancer Pain Guidelines (now Agency for Healthcare Research and Quality [AHRQ])[9]

      vi. Grassroots development of State Cancer Pain Initiatives (now American Alliance of Cancer Pain Initiatives)

      vii. Efforts of Project on Death in America, LAST ACTS Initiative, and Center to Improve the Care of the Dying[10]

      viii. Americans for Better Care of the Dying (ABCD)

      ix. Center to Advance Palliative Care (CAPC)

      x. JCAHO includes pain assessment and management as a part of the accreditation process for hospitals, home health, long-term care, long-term care pharmacies, ambulatory care, behavioral health, managed behavioral health, healthcare networks[11]

III.   Hospice Philosophy

A.   Definitions of Hospice

1. Medicare describes hospice as an approach to caring for terminally ill individuals that stresses palliative care (relief of pain and uncomfortable symptoms), as opposed to curative care. In addition to meeting the patient's medical needs, hospice care addresses the physical, psychosocial, and spiritual needs of the patient, as well as the psychosocial needs of the patient's family/caregiver. The emphasis of the hospice program is on keeping the hospice patient at home with family and friends as long as possible

2. The National Hospice and Palliative Care Organization (NHPCO) describes hospice as a specialized form of multidisciplinary healthcare which is designed to provide palliative care, alleviate the physical, emotional, social and spiritual discomforts of an individual who is experiencing the last phase of life due to the existence of a life-limiting, progressive disease, to provide supportive care to the primary caregiver and the family of the hospice patient

3. Hospice and Palliative Nurses Association (HPNA) defines hospice nursing as the provision of palliative nursing care for the terminally ill and their families with the emphasis on their physical, psychosocial, emotional, and spiritual needs. This care is accomplished in collaboration with an interdisciplinary team through a service that is available 24 hours a day, 7 days a week. The service comprises pain and symptom management, bereavement and volunteer components. Hospice nursing, then, is holistic practice conducted within an affiliated matrix. The hospice nurse, in developing and maintaining collaborative relationships with other members of the interdisciplinary team, must be flexible in dealing with the inevitable role blending that takes place. In functioning as a case manager, coordinating the implementation of the interdisciplinary team developed plan of care, the hospice nurse also shares an advocacy role for patients and their families with other members of the team

B.   Key Concepts in Hospice Philosophy

1. The patient and family (as defined by the patient) are considered the single unit of care

2. Hospice uses a core interdisciplinary team to address the physical, social, emotional and spiritual needs of the patient and family

3. Hospice provides for the medical treatment of pain and other distressing symptoms associated with the life-limiting, progressive illness, but does not provide interventions to cure the disease or prolong life

4. The interdisciplinary team develops the overall plan of care, in accordance with the wishes of the patient and family, in order to provide coordinated care that emphasizes supportive services such as home care, pain management and limited inpatient services

5. Hospice care actively engages the community by utilizing volunteer support in delivering hospice services

6. The patient's home, or place of primary residence no matter where that may be (skilled nursing or residential care facilities, prisons, shelters, daycare centers for the elderly, etc.), is the primary site of hospice care

7. The philosophy of hospice emphasizes comfort, dignity and quality of life, with the focus on spiritual and existential issues throughout dying, death and bereavement

8. Patients and families are empowered to achieve as much control over their lives as possible

C. Desired Goals for End of Life Care[12]

1. Self-determined life closure: terminally ill patients who are mentally competent should have freedom to decide how the rest of their life is spent within the options allowed by law

2. Safe and comfortable dying: patients are able to die free of distressing symptoms

3. Effective grieving: surviving family members/significant others are supported through the normal grieving process

D. Issues for Hospice

1. Six months life expectancy (should the disease run its usual course) or less may be seen as death sentence by some physicians who thus may be reluctant to refer to hospice

2. Insurers may not pay for high-tech care and may limit access to specialists

3. Physicians may be reluctant to discuss Do Not Resuscitate (DNR) orders; patient and family may not be ready to accept them although DNR orders are not required for hospice admission

4. Referrals often occur when death is imminent, thus rushing hospice to quickly bond with family and initiate symptom management in crisis mode

5. Significant barriers to the management of pain continue to exist (see Chapter IV)

IV. Philosophy of Palliative Care

A. Definitions of Palliative Care

1. The National Hospice and Palliative Care Organization (NHPCO) defined palliative care as treatment that enhances comfort and improves quality of life. No specific therapy is excluded from consideration. The test of palliative treatment lies in the agreement by the individual physician(s), primary caregiver and the hospice team that the expected outcome is relief from distressing symptoms, the easing of pain, and/or enhancing the quality of life[13]

2. World Health Organization defines palliative care as an approach to care which improves quality of life of patients and their families facing life threatening illness, through the prevention and relief of suffering by means of early identification and impeccable assessment and treatment of pain and other problems, physical, psychological and spiritual[14]

3. Canadian Palliative Care Association states palliative care is a philosophy of care that provides a combination of active and compassionate therapies intended to support and comfort individuals and families who are living with life threatening illness, being sensitive and respectful of their religious, cultural, and personal beliefs, values and traditions[15]

4. Palliative care is defined as "...the prevention and relief of suffering through the management of symptoms from the early through the final stages of an illness" and "...attends closely to the emotional, spiritual, and practical needs/goals of the patient/family with life-threatening disease across the illness, dying trajectory."[7]

5. American Acadamy of Hospice and Palliative Medicine defines palliative care as "comprehensive, specialized care provided by an interdisciplinary team to patients and families living with a life threatening or severe advanced illness expected to progress toward dying and where care is particularly focused on alleviating suffering and promoting quality of life. Major concerns are pain and symptom management, information sharing and advance care planning, psychosocial and spiritual support, and coordination of care"[16,p1]

6. Hospice and Pallaitve Nurses Assocition defines end-of-life care as nurisng care for people expereinceing life-limiting progressive illness

B. **Key Concepts of Palliative Care Philosophy**[17]

1. Affirms life and regards dying as a normal process that is neither hastened nor postponed

2. Provides relief from pain and other distressing symptoms

3. Integrates the psychological and spiritual aspects of patient care

4. Offers a support system to help the family cope during the patient's illness and their own bereavement

C. **Precepts of Palliative Care according to the Last Acts Initiative, 1998**

1. Respect for patient goals, preferences and choices

2. Comprehensive care

   a) Addresses holistic needs

   b) Alleviates isolation

   c) Commits to ongoing communication and non-abandonment

3. Utilizes strengths of interdisciplinary resources

4. Acknowledges/addresses caregiver concerns and desire for supportive services

5. Develops institutional infrastructures that support best practices and best models of palliative care

6. Excellent interdisciplinary team coordination among all caregiving environments

7. Focus of care based on patient and family values, addresses holistic growth and healing

8. Care is flexible, e.g., curative, palliative, or preventive in focus

D. **Core Principles of Palliative Care**

1. Family is the unit of care

2. Meaning of disease, suffering, life and death are addressed within each unique family unit

3. Commitment to collaboration through team process

4. Ethical principles of care are incorporated into daily practice

E. Issues for Palliative Care

1. Patients, families and staff may have difficulty transitioning from curative to palliative care

2. Most programs are located in hospital-based, hierarchical medical institutions

3. Some programs may not provide continuity and communication with primary care physicians and community-based programs

4. Some programs may not provide supportive services, such as social work, spiritual, volunteer or bereavement follow-up

Cited References

1. Conner SR. New initiatives transforming hospice care. *The Hospice Journal.* 1999;14(3/4):193–203.

2. O'Connor P. Hospice vs. palliative care. *The Hospice Journal.* 1999;14(3/4):123–137.

3. Byock IR. Hospice and palliative care: a parting of the ways or a path to the future. *Journal of Palliative Medicine.* 1998;1:165–76.

4. Portenoy PR. *Defining Palliative Care.* Beth Israel Medical Center: Newsletter, Department of Pain and Palliative Care; 1998.

5. Brenner R. Hospice care and palliative care: a perspective from experience. *The Hospice Journal.* 1999;14(3/4):155–166.

6. The SUPPORT Principal Investigators. A controlled trial to improve care for seriously ill patients. *JAMA.* 1995;274:1591–1598.

7. Field MJ, Cassel CK. *Approaching Death: Improving Care at the End of Life.* Washington, DC: Institute of Medicine Task Force: 1997.

8. World Health Organization (WHO). Report of a WHO Expert Committee *Cancer Pain Relief and Palliative Care.* WHO Technical Support Series, No. 804. Geneva: World Health Organization; 1986, 1990, 1996.

9. Jacox A, Carr DB, Payne R, et al. *Management of Cancer Pain. Clinical Practice Guideline* No. 9. AHCPR Publication No. 94-0592. Rockville, MD: Agency for Health Care Policy and Research, U.S. Department of Health and Human Services, Public Health Service; March 1994.

10. Matzo ML, Sherman DW. *Palliative Care Nursing: Quality Care to the End of Life.* New York: Springer Publishing; 2001.

11. Joint Commission on Accreditation of Healthcare Organizations. Accreditation Overviews. Available at: http://www.jcaho.org/htba/index.htm. Accessed January 25, 2005.

12. National Hospice Organization. *A Pathway for Patients and Families Facing Terminal Illness.* Arlington, VA: National Hospice Organization; 1997:5–6.

13. National Hospice and Palliative Care Organization (NHPCO). *Standards of Practice for Hospice Programs. Arlington, VA: NHPCO; 2000:ii.*

14. World Health Organization, *National Cancer Control Programs: Policies and Managerial Guidelines.* 2nd ed. 2002.

15. Canadian Palliative Care Association, *Palliative Care: Towards a Consensus in Standardized Principles of Practice.* Canadian Palliative Care Association; 1995.

16. American Academy of Hospice and Palliative Medicine. Position Statement: Definitions of Palliative Care and Palliative Medicine. Availiable at http://www.aahpm.org/positions/definition.html. Accessed March 4, 2005.

17. Storey P, Knight, CF. *Hospice/Palliative Care Training For Physicians (UNIPACS 2, 2, 4, 6).* Chicago, IL: American Academy of Hospice and Palliative Medicine; 1996 & 1997.

Additional References and Resources

Abu-Saad HH. Palliative care: An international view. *Patient Education and Counseling.* 2000; 41:15–22.

Ferrell BR, Coyle N, eds. *Textbook of Palliative Nursing.* New York, NY: Oxford University Press; 2001.

Krisman-Scott MA. Origins of hospice in the United States: the care of the dying, 1945–1975. *Journal of Hospice and Palliative Nursing.* 2002:5(4):205–210.

National Hospice and Palliative Care Organization. *Facts and Figures on Hospice Care in America.* Washington, DC: National Hospice and Palliative Care Organization; 2001.

Payne SK, et al. *A High Volume Specialist Palliative Care Unit (PCU) and Team Reduces End of Life (EOL) Costs.* American Society of Clinical Oncology; 2001.

Saunders C. The evolution of palliative care. *Patient Education and Counseling.* 2000; 41:7–13.

CHAPTER II

THE INTERDISCIPLINARY TEAM IN HOSPICE AND PALLIATIVE NURSING

Linda M. Gorman, RN, MN, APRN, BC, CHPN®, OCN

I. Introduction

A. The Interdisciplinary Team (IDT)

1. The interdisciplinary team is a group of individuals with varied and specialized training who collaborate to coordinate their activities to provide services for clients

2. In hospice and/or palliative care the IDT usually consists of the professionals and nonprofessionals who are involved in the care of the patient and his/her family

3. The complex physical, psychosocial, spiritual, and financial issues facing the patient and his/her family receiving hospice and palliative care requires professionals with a broad range of knowledge[1-3]

4. Because of the complex and multidimensional needs of seriously ill and terminally ill patients, the interdisciplinary team in hospice and palliative care is essential[1-2]

5. No one professional can address all the complex needs of these patients/families so working with a group of team members representing multiple disciplines ensures that the varied needs can be met more effectively

6. A strength of the team is that each member has a unique view of the patient/family[3]

7. In hospice, core team members required by hospice regulations include

   a) Hospice Physician

   b) RN Case Manager

   c) Social Worker

   d) Counselor

8. Other hospice team members may include other nurses, home health aides, volunteers, pharmacists, chaplains, bereavement coordinators, dietitians, psychologists, and therapists, amongst others

9. Palliative care interdisciplinary team membership is more varied but can include the following[4]

   a) Core group of professionals should include medicine, nursing (include advanced practice nurse and social work)

   b) Others may include some combination of following

      i. Volunteer coordinators

      ii. Dietitians

      iii. Nursing assistants

      iv. Pharmacists

      v. Chaplains

      vi. Bereavement coordinators

      vii. Psychologists

      viii. Therapists (physical, occupations, art, play music, child-life)

      ix. Trained volunteers

10. Each member of the team has a unique view of the patient and family[3]

11. Important components of the interdisciplinary team[1]

   a) Collaboration

   b) Patient/Family-directed goal setting

   c) Interdisciplinary planning of interventions

12. The key to effective interdisciplinary team functioning includes collaboration, leadership, coordinated decision-making, and conflict resolution[3]

B. **Multidisciplinary team**

   1. In the traditional multidisciplinary approach, members representing each discipline independently formulate goals based on their own area of expertise[5]

   2. The group may meet but independent plans from each discipline are developed

   3. In other models the group may only communicate through the medical record rather than meeting face to face

   4. The physician is often the team leader in a traditional multidisciplinary team[3]

   5. This model is often utilized in the acute hospital setting

   6. The multidisciplinary team is not utilized in the hospice/palliative care setting

II. Collaboration of the IDT

A. **Characteristics of effective collaboration[3,6]**

   1. Assessment data is shared so all disciplines have the same information

   2. All members participate in development of the plan of care

3. Information is utilized in accordance with the expressed needs and wishes of the patient and family

4. Shared planning, decision making, accountability and responsibility for the care of the patient are implied in the interdisciplinary team

5. Collaboration implies that team members are aware of each other's roles. This can be accomplished by

    a) Joint visits so disciplines can understand each other's contributions

    b) Educating team members of role functions

    c) All team members respect and attend to assessments and contributions made by each other

    d) Team members understand their own role in the team and appreciation of the contribution of other members is fostered

6. Team members must collaborate with other healthcare professionals essential to the patient's care who may not be part of the interdisciplinary team e.g., primary physician, psychotherapist, nurse practitioner from the community

7. Decisions are made after all information has been gathered and all team members contribute

8. Remaining clear on the goals for the patient and family should drive all decisions rather than one team member's perspective

9. Collaboration builds interdisciplinary awareness of interdependence of the team[1]

III. Team Leadership

A. Designating the team leader

1. Though one individual may be designated as the leader, all members share responsibility to participate and contribute

2   The team leader may be any member of the team

B. Characteristics of an effective leader of an interdisciplinary team include[6]

1. Promotes collaboration and communication

2. Encourages input from all members of the team

3. Recognizes when conflict is occurring and works with whole team to address

4. Recognizes need to complete tasks within set time-frame and works with group to accomplish this

5. Supports diverse opinions and new ideas to be introduced to the group

IV. **Coordinated Decision Making**

    A. **Team members incorporate each discipline's assessment of the patient/family into the comprehensive plan of care**[1]

    B. **Care goals are based on team member assessments and patient/family needs and wishes**

    C. **Other healthcare providers who are not part of the team will be incorporated as needed**

    D. **Team members discuss complex situations so all information is gathered before difficult decisions are made**

    E. **The plan of care is systematically updated on a regular basis to ensure goals defined by the patient and family are being addressed and continuity of care is maintained**

V. **Conflict Resolution**[6-7]

    A. **Communication is the foundation of all team functioning**

    B. **Conflict tends to arise when there are barriers to effective communication**

    C. **Conflict is expected to occur since members are interdependent on each other**

    D. **Team members need to feel they are equals and that each can offer ideas and recommendations on ways to improve team functioning**

    E. **Factors that may contribute to conflict within the team include**
        1. Ambiguous role boundaries
        2. Communication barriers
        3. Leadership style that is not appropriate for the situation or congruent with the team's needs
        4. Team members with differing goals and expectations
        5. Poorly stated purpose of the meeting
        6. Lack of training in interdisciplinary collaboration
        7. Group that is too large or too small for the stated purpose
        8. Poor mechanisms to achieve timely exchange of information

    F. **Types of conflict**
        1. Intrapersonal—team members may have conflicting feelings with a colleague
        2. Interpersonal—recurring differences between team members with different personality styles

      3.   Intragroup—subgroups within a team that are in conflict with other subgroups

      4.   Intergroup—conflict between programs or other teams

G. Preventing team conflict

    1.   Self awareness within team of potential conflict areas

    2.   Reviewing decisions when disagreement is evident

    3.   Examination of overlapping roles and considering renegotiation of roles and assignments

    4.   Recognize professional hierarchies exist and discuss openly e.g., some member(s) tend to defer to an experienced, well respected physician

    5.   Team building exercises

    6.   Develop ground rules

    7.   Encourage open environment to discuss disagreements

    8.   Invite other professionals to the team meeting and encourage their input

    9.   Develop an evaluation process of team functioning that is accomplished periodically

   10. Analyze retention rates and satisfaction levels of members

H. Addressing team conflict

    1.   Most important is to recognize team conflict and not ignore it

    2.   Brainstorm possible solutions with whole team

    3.   Separate the person from the problem e.g., avoid focusing on an individual's personality trait that irritates some members. Rather focus on how the trait impacts communication

    4.   Use objective criteria when possible

    5.   Seek outside consultation with organizational development professionals when needed

    6.   Support constructive and respectful criticism

    7.   Identify areas of agreement

    8.   Remember that the presence of conflict can often bring growth and potential for change and should not be avoided[3]

VI. LP/VN Roles in the Interdisciplinary Team[8-9]

A. The LP/VN plays an important role in the IDT

    1.   Communicate information from systematic data collection of the multidimensional aspects of the needs of the patients and family

    2.   Collaborate with other members of the interdisciplinary team

    3.   Participate in the development of the individualized plan of care

    4.   Address conflicts through appropriate institutional policies and procedures and other resources

5.   Demonstrate professional accountability

6   Facilitate open discussion with health team members about the patient/family concerns

7.   Participate in team meetings

8.   Collaborates with patient and family

VII. Additional Members of the Interdisciplinary Team[3]

A.   Hospice/Palliative Care Physician

1.   Primary function is to consult with primary care physician and collaborate with hospice/palliative care team on management of patient's symptoms

2.   Relies on the nurses who generally have more prolonged contact with the patient to provide important assessment information

3.   Collaborates with all team members

B.   Registered Nurse

1.   Completes the assessment of the patient and family and supervises other nursing personnel seeing the patient including the LP/VN and nurses aide

2.   Communicates assessment information and interventions

3.   Collaborates with all team members

C.   Social Worker

1.   Assesses strengths and resources of the patient/family system and implements interventions including emotional support

2.   Provides resources to patient/families

3.   Collaborates with all team members

D.   Spiritual Counselor

1.   Completes in-depth assessment of patient/family spiritual needs

2.   Acts as liaison with community clergy when needed

3.   Acts as a resource to the team on spiritual questions as well as participating in the development of the plan of care

4.   Collaborates with all team members

VIII. Characteristics of a Well-Functioning Hospice and/or Palliative Care Team[5-6,10-12]

A.   Members willingness to take professional risks e.g., share personal limitations, recognize need to get help from others

B.   Members display trust amongst each other e.g., able to share mistakes

C.   Successes and failures are shared

D.   Contributions of all members are acknowledged

E.   Information shared in the team setting remains confidential and is not shared inappropriately outside of the meeting

F.   There is recognition of when a team member needs assistance

G.   Shared leadership activities can be a function of trust

H.   Majority of members attend most meetings

I.   Each member participates actively in the care planning process

J.   Members treat each other with respect

K.   Members seek out opinion of other members

L.   Patients and families express satisfaction with the care provided by the team

M.   Positive patient outcomes have traditionally been viewed as reflecting an effective team

N.   Patient and family remain at the center

O.   Changes in membership do not cause a major shift in outcomes

IX. Evaluation Process of the Interdisciplinary Team Functions[6-7]

A.   Monitoring performance improvement indicators

B.   Evaluating patient/family satisfaction

C.   Exit interviews when team members leave

D.   Periodic surveys of members to express concerns

CITED REFERENCES

1   Egan KA, Labyak MJ. Hospice care: a model for quality end-of-life care. In: Ferrell BR, Coyle N. eds. *Textbook of Palliative Nursing.* New York: Oxford University Press; 2001:7–26.

2. Center for Advancement of Palliative Care. Recruiting an Interdisciplinary Team. Available at www.old.capc.org/topic/11/. Accessed July 12, 2004.

3. Krammer LM, Ring AA, Martinez J, Jacobs MJ, Williams MB. The nurse's role in interdisciplinary and palliative care. In: Matzo ML, Sherman DW, eds. *Palliative Nursing Care: Quality Care to the End of Life.* New York, NY: Springer Publishing; 2001:118–139.

4. National Consensus Project. Clinical Practice Guidelines for Quality Palliative Care. Available at www.nationalconsensusproject.org. Accessed July 20, 2004.

5. Geriatric Interdisciplinary Team Training Curriculum. Topic 1:Teams and Teamwork. Available at www.gitt.org. Accessed June 26, 2004.

6. Lynn J, Schuster JL, Kabcenel A. *Improving Care for the End of Life.* New York, NY: Oxford University Press; 2000.

7. Geriatric Interdisciplinary Team Training Curriculum. Topic 3: Team Communication and Conflict Resolution. Available at www.gitt.org. Accessed June 26, 2004.

8. Dahlin C, Lentz J, Sutermaster DJ. *Professional Competencies for the Hospice and Palliative Licensed Practical/Vocational Nurse.* Dubuque, IA: Kendall/Hunt Publishing; 2004.

9. Dahlin C, Lentz J, Sutermaster DJ. *Statement on the Scope and Standards of Hospice and Palliative Licensed Practical/Vocational Nursing Practice.* Dubuque, IA: Kendall/Hunt Publishing; 2004.

10. Temkin-Greener H, Gross D, Kunitz SJ, Mukamel D. Measuring interdisciplinary team performance in a long-term care setting. *Medical Care.* 2004;42(5):472–481.

11. Stevenson L. The role and function of the interdisciplinary psychotherapeutic team in oncology care. In: Carroll-Johnson RM, Gorman LM, Bush NJ, eds. *Psychosocial Nursing Along the Cancer Continuum.* Pittsburgh, PA: ONS Press; 1998:277–284.

12. McKenna RJ, Russel C. *Cancer Rehabilitation: A Team Approach for the Community Hospital.* Sacramento, CA: American Cancer Society; 1984.

ADDITIONAL REFERENCES AND RESOURCES

Cartwright J, Kayser-Jones J. End-of-life care in assisted living facilities: perceptions of residents, families and staffs. *Journal of Hospice and Palliative Nursing.* 2002:5(3):143–151.

Egan KA, Abbott P. Interdisciplinary team training: preparing new employees for the specialty of hospice and palliative care. *Journal of Hospice and Palliative Nursing.* 2002:4(3):153–160.

Lovelady B, Sword T. Hospice care planning: an interdisciplinary roadmap. *Journal of Hospice and Palliative Nursing.* 2002:6(4):223–231.

Mazanec P, Bartel J, Buras D, Fessler P, Hudson J. Jacoby M, Montana B, Phillips M. Transdisciplinary pain management: a holistic approach. *Journal of Hospice and Palliative Nursing.* 2002:4(4):228–234.

CHAPTER III

PATTERNS OF DISEASE PROGRESSION

Bev Paukstis, RN, MS, CHPN®

Adapted from: Dahlin C, Kalina K. Patterns of Disease Progression.
In: Volker BG, Watson AC, eds. *Core Curriculum for the Generalist Hospice and Palliative Nurse.*
Kendall/Hunt Publishing: Dubuque, IA; 2002:29–61.

I.   **Cancer**

   A   **Definition: Cancer is a disease of the cells. In this disease cells lose their normal controls and traits. The disease causes the cells to have unregulated growth, lack of differentiation, and provides cells with the ability to invade local tissues and then spread to other organs. This cell growth is named "tumor." The word "oncology" means the scientific study of tumors. *Onco* is derived from the Greek word *onkos* which means mass or tumor**

   B.   **Cancer is the second leading cause of death in the United States[1]**

   C.   **Major cancer diagnoses**

      1.   Lung cancer

         a)   Symptoms: cough, hemoptysis, dyspnea, pneumonia, pain in the shoulder or arm

         b)   Common metastatic sites: brain, bone, liver

         c)   Psychosocial issues: guilt about smoking, fear of suffocating

      2.   Breast cancer

         a)   Symptoms: painless mass in the breast, dimpling of skin of breast, nipple changes, one breast is different from the other, change in texture of the skin, discharge of any kind from the nipple, scaling of skin of areola or nipple

         b)   Common metastatic sites: bone, liver, brain, lung

         c)   Psychosocial issues: fears over losses of femininity, sexuality; perception of body as being abnormal

3. Reproductive cancers

   a) Ovarian cancer

      i. Symptoms: increased abdominal girth, changes in bowel patterns, weight loss, vague complaints of nausea, palpable mass (in advanced stage)

      ii. Common metastatic sites: lung, liver, peritoneal linings

      iii. Diagnosis usually occurs late in the disease process death most likely due to the GI complications being treated symptomatically only

      iv. Genetic predisposition; tumor marker study CA-25 is recommended for prediction of disease and its presence

      v. Psychosocial issues: anger with medical system due to late diagnosis, fear of death, sexual dysfunction

   b) Endometrial cancer

      i. Symptoms: changes in bowel patterns, vaginal bleeding, jaundice, ascites, dyspnea

      ii. Common metastatic sites: bone, peritoneal linings

      iii. Psychosocial issues: sexual dysfunction, frustration with treatment that is rarely helpful

   c) Cervical cancer

      i. Symptoms: associated with metastasis to bladder because disease is not diagnosed until late in the process: dysuria, urinary retention, urinary frequency, hematuria; rectal bleeding, changes in bowel patterns

      ii. Common metastatic sites: bladder, bone, GU system

      iii. Psychosocial issues: guilt over failure to obtain PAP smears, guilt over sexual habits (Herpes II and human papillomavirus [HPV] are precursors), sexuality

   d) Testicular cancer

      i. Symptoms are not seen until late in the disease: back pain, bone pain (due to probable metastases to bone), dyspnea, seizures, headache, cough (due to probable metastasis to lung, brain)

      ii. Common metastatic sites: bone, lung, liver

      iii. Psychosocial issues: some clinicians and researchers have linked with high use of certain sports such as biking and baseball

      iv. Despite metastasis and advanced disease, usually curable

4. Genitourinary cancers

   a) Prostate cancer

      i. Symptoms initially are difficulty in urinating and hematuria progressing to painful defecation, weight loss and worsening urinary obstruction

      ii. Common metastatic sites: bone, most often the bone pain is the patient's chief complaint

b) Bladder cancer

  i.   Symptoms: hematuria, flank pain, changes in urination function (dysuria, frequency, urgency), renal failure

  ii. Common metastatic sites: GU system, peritoneal linings

  iii. Psychosocial issues: potential for loss of sexuality when surgery is done; males may become impotent and in females the anterior wall of the vagina may be removed

c) Kidney cancer

  i.   Symptoms: gross hematuria, dull pain, palpable abdominal mass, fever, weight loss, dyspnea, anemia

  ii. Common metastatic sites: bone, lung, liver, brain

  iii. Psychosocial issues: guilt over cigarette smoking; there is a possible link to exposure to asbestos, cadmium and lead

5. Gastrointestinal cancers

a) Colon, rectal and anal cancers

  i.   Symptoms: constipation, incontinence, weight loss, sensation of rectal fullness, dull perineal or sacral pain radiating down legs, rectal bleeding

  ii. Common metastatic sites: lung, liver

  iii. Psychosocial issues: guilt over incurring what is now seen as preventable; potential for distortion of body image due to a colostomy

b) Esophageal cancer

  i.   Symptoms: dysphasia, signs of airway obstruction, dehydration, general debilitation

  ii. Diagnosis most often occurs in advanced stages of disease, very poor prognosis

  iii. Common metastatic sites: lung, liver, adrenal glands

  iv. Psychosocial issues: disease usually grows rapidly

c) Pancreatic cancer

  i.   Symptoms: extreme jaundice, abdominal pain, nausea, vomiting, diarrhea, feeling of fullness, bloating

  ii. Common metastatic sites: lung, liver bowel, rectum

  iii. Psychosocial issues: depression frequently accompanies this diagnosis more than other cancer diagnoses. Believed to be correlated with sugar metabolism

d) Gastric cancer (stomach)

  i.   Symptoms: weight loss, malnutrition, weakness

  ii. Common metastatic sites: lung, liver, bowel, rectum

  iii. Psychosocial issues: in most cultures, food equals caring and often caregiver— patient stress occurs over inability to eat

e) Liver

    i.   Symptoms: bloating, weight loss, pain, bleeding, nausea, vomiting, jaundice, anorexia, itching of skin (pruritus), peripheral edema, confusion

    ii.   Common metastatic sites: bone, lung

    iii.   Psychosocial issues: may be associated with cirrhosis (alcoholic or nutritional) hence possible guilt over prevention; aggressive disease

6.   Leukemia/malignant blood disorders

   a)   Leukemia

    i.   Disorder of blood and the organs that make blood resulting in uncontrolled growth of white blood cells[2]

    ii.   Symptoms; easy and frequent bruising, nose bleeds, bleeding from gums, bladder or bowel, general malaise, fever, frequent infections

    iii.   Common metastatic sites; bone, bone marrow, skin, lung, brain

    iv.   Psychosocial issues: remission and relapse cycles cause emotional fatigue; occurs frequently in children

   b)   Multiple Myeloma

    i.   Is a tumor of the plasma cells of the blood resulting in malignant masses of plasma cells spread out in the bones and tissues[2]

    ii.   Symptoms: persistent and unexplained skeletal pain, recurrent bacterial infections, anemia, pathologic fractures, constipation, renal failure

    iii.   Psychosocial issues: there may be long periods of remission leading to false hope of total cure

   c)   Lymphoma

    i.   Is a group of malignant growths that arises in the connective tissue and the lymphatic system may be secondary to patients with AIDS

    ii.   Symptom: fever, night sweats, weight loss, itching, low back pain, shortness of breath, decreased urinary output

    iii.   Common metastatic sites: bone, bone marrow, skin, lung, brain

7.   Melanoma

   a)   Is a tumor growing in a pigmented area of skin

   b)   Symptoms: a visible lesion with varieties of size, color, shape, and growth habit

   c   Common metastatic sites: bone, lung, liver, brain

   d)   Psychosocial issues: guilt over possible prevention, distortion of body image secondary to tumors or surgery

8. Head and Neck cancers

    a) Symptoms: pain, visible lesions and tumors in mouth, neck, head; pain, ulcerated areas

    b) Common metastatic sites: skin, lung

    c) Psychosocial issues: distortion of self-image, depression, social isolation, possible inability to speak due to tracheostomy

9. Brain tumor

    a) Symptoms: drowsiness, decreased attention span, mood changes, poor judgment, impaired cognitive skills, short term memory loss, headache, vomiting, irregularities of heart rate, seizures, personality changes, malnutrition, dehydration, hiccoughs

    b) Common metastatic site: the meninges of the brain

    c) Psychosocial issues: has often been termed "lesions of the spirit" because of the ways in which mental status is attacked and altered

II. Treatment of Cancer

A. Surgery

1. Removal of tumor

2. Can be curative: all tumor and a margin of surrounding tissues are removed

3. Can be palliative: tumor is removed as much as possible to lessen pain and symptoms

B. Radiation Therapy

1. Use of radiation to remove cells in localized cancer treatment. May be curative for some cancers

2. Use of radiation to treat tissues or organs before the disease clinically evident

3. Promote the eradication of cells causing distressing symptoms. May be palliative for oncologic emergencies such as spinal cord compression or superior vena cava syndrome

C. Chemotherapy

1. Is the administration of medication specifically made to destroy the cells of tumors

2. Treats cancer in 3 ways

    a) Cure: alone or with radiation and/or surgery

    b) Control: used to extend life when cure is not possible

    c) Palliate: used to relieve the distress of some symptoms and pain when neither cure nor control is possible; e.g., decrease of bowel tumor size so that stool can pass

3. Side effects[3]

    a) Short-term: (few days): nausea, vomiting, stomatitis, diarrhea, anorexia long term: peripheral nerve damage with resulting peripheral neuropathies and pain—constipation, toxicity to kidneys, toxicity to heart, hemorrhagic bladder infection (cystitis), pulmonary fibrosis, clinically evident

D. Supportive and Alternative Treatments

1. Blood transfusions, artificial nutrition administration (tube feedings, TPN)

2. Complementary therapies of vitamin and herbal supplements, psychological techniques, support groups

III. Human Immunodeficiency Virus Infection (HIV Infection)

A. Definition: HIV is a group of retroviruses that invade a host cell's DNA and this results in a wide range of clinical presentations varying from no symptoms to fever, debilitation and fatal related disorders

B. Transmission requires close contact with body fluids

1. Contaminated blood products

2. Sexual contact: rectal, vaginal

3. Organ transplant and insemination from infected donors

4. Prenatal and perinatal exposure for newborns (pregnancy, childbirth, breastfeeding)

5. Occupational injuries such as needle sticks, sharps sticks. Sharing of contaminated needles by IV drug users

C. Can be managed with retroviral drugs

D. Cluster of symptoms: malaise, fatigue, weight loss, intermittent fever, chronic diarrhea, lymphadenopathy

IV. Acquired Immunodeficiency Syndrome (AIDS)

A. Definition: infection with HIV that leads to the development of opportunistic infections and/or certain secondary cancers such as Kaposi's sarcoma and non-Hodgkin's lymphoma, and neurological dysfunction

B. Symptoms

1. Neurologic: seizures, focal motor sensory or gait disturbances, headache, lethargy

2. Infections: pneumonia, meningitis, encephalitis, thrush

C. Psychosocial issues: social isolation, depression, fear of death, guilt over possible prevention, anger. Issues related to disenfranchisement

D. Neither HIV nor AIDS can be cured. HIV can be maintained and held in check with retroviral medications. AIDS requires treatment of symptoms; it cannot be controlled or held in check

E. AIDS occurs when people cannot tolerate or do not take retroviral medications for HIV infection

F. Special grief issues in AIDS bereavement care

    1.   These issues surface for the patient in the category of anticipatory grief

        a)   Stigma of AIDS and HIV leads to social isolation

        b)   Stigma of substance abuse

        c)   Guilt over behaviors that may be causes

    2.   These issues may surface for members of the family or origin and friends

        a)   Homophobia

        b)   Multiple losses

        c)   Disenfranchised grief

V. **Neurological Conditions**

A. **Causes**

    1.   Injury (internal)

        a)   Cerebrovascular accident (CVA)—3rd leading cause of deaths in USA, resulting in death of brain cells due to clots (embolism) in a blood vessel, rupture in a vessel or of an aneurysm, or due to the presence of plaque in the cerebral blood vessels, damage depends on location and size

    2.   Injury (external)

        a)   Trauma to skull

        b)   Intracranial or subdural bleeding and prolonged pressure within the brain and skull leads to damages similar to CVA

    3.   Degenerative Diseases

        a)   Amyotrophic Lateral Sclerosis (ALS)—a motor neuron disease in the cerebral cortex, the brainstem, the spinal cord. Results in progressive weakness and atrophy of muscles. Usually there is no change in mentation

        b)   Dementia—Alzheimer's or other type—an irreversible and progressive dementia characterized by mentation deterioration, disorganization of personality, results in total inability to execute any daily living tasks including eating

    c)   Parkinson's Disease—idiopathic, slowly progressing degenerative disorder of the CNS characterized by slow movements, muscle rigidity, resting tremor and postural instability

B. Treatment

1. Medications to relieve the symptoms, such as steroids for injuries to the brain

2. ALS and Alzheimer's disease have trials of drugs in process

3. Functional care focuses on re-establishing or maintaining ADLs, providing appropriate nutrition, preventing complications related to being immobile

4. Psychosocial support to patient and to family

C. Consideration in Advanced Disease

1. Injury: permanent neurological damage predisposes to complications: dysphasia, incontinence, infections. Death is usually related to subsequent CVAs or major infection

2. Degenerative diseases: progressive weakness, dysphasia, respiratory diminishment, infections and seizures as well as immobility all contribute to the dying process

VI. Cardiac Conditions

This category includes diseases of the heart which cause damage to the heart muscle through various mechanisms, that result in loss of oxygen to the heart or decreased cardiac output

A. Causes

1. Half of the cases are idiopathic (unknown cause)

2. The rest can be the result of chronic high alcohol intake, inherited tendencies, metabolic and endocrine diseases, infection, and coronary artery disease

B. Treatment

1. Surgical: heart transplant, angioplasty, bypass surgery

2. Pharmacologic: diuretics, nitrates, morphine, calcium channel blockers, beta blockers, ACE inhibitors, vasodilators, glycosides

3. Cardiac rehab, diet changes, stress management

C. Advanced Disease

1. Congestive heart failure (CHF): failure of the heart to be able to function properly due to an accumulation of situations that prevent adequate performance. These are conditions that no longer or never could respond to treatment modalities

2. Symptoms of congestive heart failure: anxiety, restlessness, dyspnea, tachycardia, palpitations, lung wheezes, fatigue, cyanosis or pallor, dependent peripheral edema, weight gain, cough, hemoptysis

3. Psychosocial issue: inability to resolve impending death due to success of previous rescue efforts through drugs or CPR/ventilator

VII. Pulmonary Diseases

A. Lung Diseases Are Either Obstructive or Restrictive

1. Obstructive (chronic obstructive pulmonary disease—COPD): small airways have chronic spasms cause by disease, tobacco, toxins

    a) Emphysema—damage to the airways due to elastin breakdown which causes a decreased ability of alveolar to expel air. Dyspnea is the result of air trapped in the aveoli.[4] Symptoms

    i. Patient has muscle wasting progressive external dyspnea

    ii. Accessory muscles are used for breathing

    iii. Chest is "barrel" in appearance, patient cannot cough well, breath sounds are weak

    b) Chronic bronchitis—increased secretion of thick 'sticky' mucous that increases risk of pulmonary infections. Chronic cough is the result of mucous and is difficult to clear due to damaged cilia and thickened inflamed bronchial walls.[4] Symptoms

    i. Patient is overweight

    ii. Cyanosis is present

    iii. Breath is wheezing

2. Restrictive: loss of lung tissues which causes limited lung expansion due to other diseases such as cancer, fibrosis, and myasthenia gravis

B. Treatment

1. For COPD: pharmacologic (bronchodilators, corticosteroids, xanthenes, anticholinergics), oxygen

2. For restricted lung disease: pharmacologic (corticosteroids, nebulizers/IPPB), oxygen

C. Advanced Disease

1. Both types of lung disease eventually result in lung failure

2. Management of symptoms is focused on comfort

    a) Medication regimens that are supplemented by anti-anxiety agents and morphine

    b) Mechanisms and techniques that promote calm: massage, imaging, hypnosis, relaxation, purse lip breathing

D. Psychosocial issues: guilt over lifestyles that may have caused disease and fear of suffocation

VIII. Kidney Diseases

A. **The inability of kidneys to function is called "renal failure." The causes include toxins, some medications, tumors, infections, diabetes, hypertension, collagen vascular diseases such as lupus or scleroderma**

B. **Treatment**

1. Dialysis: peritoneal or hemodialysis is useful in short term renal failure when the kidneys are expected to resume function; may also be used long-term when there is no expectation of return of kidney function

2. Surgery: debulking of tumors, insertion of nephrostomy tubes

3. Pharmacologic: diuretics, dietary management, treatment of underlying causes such as antihypertensives

4. Nutrition: focuses on low sodium, low protein, low potassium foods

C. **Advanced Disease**

1. Fluid and electrolyte imbalance, anemia, uremia

2. Treatment is focused on comfort through medication

3. Psychosocial issues: most compelling is the decision to continue or stop dialysis

IX. General Debility

A. **Debility, unspecified, is now a diagnostic category for elderly and debilitated persons with functional disabilities and progressive multiple organ failure who do not meet the criteria specific for other terminal diseases. This diagnosis takes the place of the pediatric "failure to thrive" which was used for this condition**

B. **Performance Scales**

1. Karnofsky Performance Scale (KPS)[5]

   a) 0 to 100 scale used to rate a patient's ability to do their own activities of daily living

   b) The higher the rating the less care needed

2. EGOC Performance Status[6]

   a) 0 to 5 scale used to assess how a patient's disease is effecting their ability to do activities of daily living

   b) The lower the rating, the less restrictions

3. Palliative Performance Scale (PPSv2)[7]

   a) 0% to 100% scale of five areas to communicate a patient's current level of functioning. The areas are ambulation, activity and evidence of disease, self-care, intake and conscious level

   b) The higher the score, the more independent

C. **Symptoms**

   1. Severe deficits in ADLs

   2. Poor performance scale rating

   3. Signs and symptoms of multiple organ failure

   4. Progressive physical deterioration

D. **Treatment**

   1. Symptom management

   2. Appropriate nutrition

   3. Prevention of complications

E. **Advanced disease treatment is focused on comfort through medications and provision of personal care**

X. **Endocrine Diseases**

A. **Diabetes Mellitus (DM): a group of disorders distinguished by chronic hyperglycemia, difficulties of carbohydrate, fat and protein metabolism[8]; leading cause of kidney failure.**

   1. Type 1—almost complete loss of insulin production by the B-cells of the islet of Langerhans in the pancreas. Commonly diagnosed in children. Initial symptoms include weight loss and increased thirst, hunger and urination from the lack of insulin to transport glucose into the cells. Without glucose entering the cells, the body will loose weight prompting feelings of polyphagia. The excess glucose is excreted by the kidneys which takes a large amount of water with it resulting in polyuria. After the loss of the water the body wants to drink more fluids resulting in polydipsia. Treatment includes insulin injections, a diet tailored to meet the individual's needs usually with a calorie restriction and close monitoring of blood glucose level[8]

   2. Type 2—cells become resistant to insulin which results in high levels of insulin in the blood that cannot transport glucose into the cells. Seen in mostly in adults. Symptoms are not always specific but can include being overweight, lipid disturbances and hypertension. Treatment can include weight control, diet with reduced calories, medications and close monitoring of blood glucose levels. There are multiple antidiabetic medications that can increase insulin secretion, decrease glucose production and aid cells in accepting the insulin[8]

   3. Other causes of hyperglycemia—gestational diabetes, impaired glucose tolerance as well as pancreatic injury, infection and cancer. These causes may result in diabetes mellitus[8]

B. **Treatment is directed toward maintaining control of blood sugar through insulin, oral antidiabetic drugs, diet, blood sugar monitoring and patient teaching**

C.   **Advanced disease**

    1.   Failure to adhere to control regimen can result in death at any time

    2.   Complications of DM; peripheral vascular disease, coronary artery disease, diabetic neuropathy, kidney failure, infections, impaired wound healing

D.   **Treatment focuses on comfort through the use of medications**

E.   **Psychosocial issues: anger directed toward patient by family for the perceived failure to adhere to a control regimen**

CITED REFERENCES

1. Centers for Disease Control and Prevention: National Center for Health Statistics. National Vital Statistics Report. Available at http://www.cdc.gov/nchs/data/dvs/nvsr52_09p9.pdf. Accessed February 28, 2005.

2. Mansen TJ, McCance KL. Alterations in leukocyte, lymphoid and hemostatic function. In: McCance KL, Huether SE, eds. *Pathophysiology: The Biological Basis for Disease in Adults and Children.* St. Louis, MO: Mosby; 2002:865–899.

3. Yarbo CH, Frogge MH, Goodman M, Gronwald S, eds. *Cancer Nursing Principles and Practice.* 5th ed. Sudbury, MA: Jones and Bartlett; 2000.

4. Brashers VL. Alterations in pulmonary function. In: McCance KL, Huether SE, eds. *Pathophysiology: The Biological Basis for Disease in Adults and Children.* St. Louis, MO: Mosby; 2002:1105–1144.

5. Karnofsky Performance Scale Index. Available at http://www.hospicepatients.org/karnofsky.html. Accessed February 23, 2005.

6. Eastern Cooperative Oncology Group. ECOG Performance Status. Available at http://www.ecog.org/general/perf_stat.html. Accessed February 23, 2005.

7. Victoria Hospice Society. Palliative Performance Scale (PPSv2). Available at http://palliative.info/resource_material/PPSv2.pdf. Accessed February 23, 2005.

8. Jones RE, Huether SE. Alterations in hormonal regulation. In: McCance KL, Huether SE, eds. *Pathophysiology: The Biological Basis for Disease in Adults and Children.* St. Louis, MO: Mosby; 2002:624–669.

ADDITIONAL REFERENCES AND RESOURCES

Ahya SN, Flood L, Paranjothi S, eds. *The Washington Manual of Medical Therapeutics.* St. Louis, MO: Washington University School of Medicine; 2001.

Ciezki JP, Komurcu S, Macklis R. Palliative radiotherapy. *Seminars in Oncology.* 2002;27(1):90–93.

Doyle D, Hanks GWC, Cherny NI, Calman K, eds. *Oxford Textbook of Palliative Medicine.* 3rd ed. New York, NY: Oxford University Press; 2003.

Ferrell BR, Coyle N, eds. *Textbook of Palliative Nursing.* Oxford University Press: New York; 2001:467–500.

Langford R, Thompson J, eds. *Mosby's Handbook of Diseases.* St. Louis, MO: Mosby; 2000.

CHAPTER IV

PAIN MANAGEMENT

Lynda Gruenewald-Schmitz, MSN, RN, CHPN®

Adapted from: Berry PH, Paice JA. Patient care: pain management.
In: Volker BG, Watson AC, eds. *Core Curriculum for the Generalist Hospice and Palliative Nurse.*
Dubuque, IA: Kendall/Hunt Publishing Company; 2002:63–87.

I. **Introduction**

   A. **Overview**

      1. Prevalence

         a) Pain is experienced by 70 to 90% of patients with advanced disease, 40–50% of patients experience moderate pain, and 25–30% have severe pain

         b) Pain scores (on a 0–10 scale) greater than or equal to "5" greatly impact on quality of life

      2. It is estimated that almost all patients (85–90%) could be free of pain and 98–99% pain controlled using the knowledge and tools currently available; the remaining 1–2% of patients at end of life can be offered palliative sedation (defined as providing relief of refractory and intolerable symptoms with the use of sedatives at the end of life) in addition to analgesics

         a) This practice is within the realm of good supportive palliative care and is <u>not</u> euthanasia. The goal of sedation is to relieve distress from unrelenting physical, psychological or spiritual symptoms

         b) This was formerly referred to as "terminal sedation," however this term led to confusion, suggesting assisted suicide, and the preferred terminology is palliative sedation

   B. **Barriers to both the assessment and the treatment of pain**

      1. Barriers from the patient/family perspective

         a) "Good" patients don't complain

         b) Pain is inevitable with aging

c) Strong medicine only comes in injectable form

d) Bearing the pain is better than bearing the side effects of pain medicine

e) Addiction to pain medicine is common

f) Strong pain medicine should only be used for very severe pain

g) Morphine is a "last ditch drug" used only when one is imminently dying

h) Fear of disease getting worse

2. Barriers from the nurse and physician perspective

a) The patient's self report of pain is not believed—healthcare professionals are the best judge of pain

b) In the hospital setting, pain is often not seen as important as other indicators

c) Only opioids are effective in severe pain

d) Opioids cause respiratory depression

e) Double effect: an ethical principle that permits an action, intended to have a good effect, when there is a risk of also causing a harmful effect, ONLY when the intention was to produce the good effect

   i. Double effect, as a principle guiding care, is complex, but nonetheless erroneously applied to end-of-life care, especially pain and symptom management

   ii. Adequately controlling symptoms at end of life is not known to shorten life

   iii. An analysis of the potential benefits of a therapy weighed against the possible risks should be conducted when considering any therapy

f) The confusion over addiction/tolerance/physical dependence (see below)

g) General lack of education relating to pain assessment, treatment and pharmacology in basic and graduate education programs

   i. There are still physicians and nurses who believe that morphine kills patients

   ii. There is a lack of knowledge regarding the treatment of chronic versus acute pain

3. Other barriers that impact on reporting pain and using analgesics

a) Anti-drug, "opio-phobic" culture—"Just say 'no' to drugs"

b) Restrictions that vary by state, including triplicate prescription laws or other programs that monitor provider prescribing patterns, lack of laws facilitating pain management in end-stage illness, including partial filling of scheduled medications (fractioning)

C. Important definitions

1. Pain: pain is whatever the experiencing person says it is, existing whenever he/she says it does.[1] History is 80% of the diagnosis—the patient's subjective report of pain is even more important to an accurate diagnosis, as there are no physical exam techniques or diagnostic tests to confirm pain history—*the patient's report must be accepted!*

2. Addiction: overwhelming involvement with obtaining and using a drug for its psychic benefits; not for medical reason; behavior is compulsive and subject to relapse; *quality of life is not improved or enhanced; use continues despite harm*

3. Tolerance: after repeated administration of an opioid, a given dosage begins to lose its effectiveness; first in duration of action; second in overall effectiveness. Dose should be gradually titrated upward to maintain the opioid's effectiveness

4. Analgesic Ceiling: a dose beyond which additional analgesic effect is not obtained

5. Physical Dependence: after repeated administration of an opioid, withdrawal symptoms occur when the drug is not taken

   a) Signs and symptoms of abstinence syndrome (withdrawal) include anxiety, irritability, lacrimation, rhinorrhea, sweating, nausea, vomiting, cramps, insomnia, and *rarely* multifocal myoclonus

   b) Appearance of abstinence syndrome is a function of the elimination half-life of the opioid; for example, abstinence symptoms appear between 6–12 hours and peak between 24–72 hours following the last dose of a medication with a short half-life (morphine is an example)

   c) Conversely, with medications with a longer half-life, the appearance of abstinence symptoms are delayed, for example, with methadone, as much as 36 to 48 hours

6. Opioid "pseudo-addiction": an iatrogenic syndrome in which patients develop certain behavioral characteristics of psychological dependence as a consequence of inadequate pain treatment[2,3]

7. Palliative Care: active total treatment and care of patients whose disease is not responsive to curative treatment. Control of pain, other symptoms, and of psychological, social, and spiritual problems is paramount. The goal of palliative care is achievement of the best possible quality of life for patients and their families. Many aspects of palliative care are also applicable earlier in the course of the illness, in conjunction with anticancer treatment. Palliative care encompasses several different settings where terminal patients receive their care including hospice and home health settings, long-term care facilities and acute care hospitals. Palliative care utilizes a team approach[4]

II. Assessment of Pain—Effectiveness of Pain Management Is Directly Related to Assessment

A. Types of Pain

1. Acute pain: usually clear cause; meaningful; perceived as reversible; observable signs (such as increased pulse rate, increase in blood pressure; nonverbal signs and symptoms, such as facial expressions, tense muscles); examples: myocardial infarction, acute appendicitis

2. Chronic or persistent: often not a clear cause; does not fulfill a useful purpose; perceived as irreversible; cyclical (aching—agony); decreased social interaction, insomnia, depressed affect; few observable or behavioral signs; examples: cancer pain, chronic back pain

3. Nociceptive pain (or somatic and visceral pain) arises from direct stimulation of the afferent nerves due to tumor infiltration, of skin, soft tissue, or viscera

    a) Somatic pain: well-localized; often described as deep, dull ache; musculoskeletal in nature

        i.   Examples: bone metastasis, inflammation of soft tissue, tumor invasion of soft tissue

        ii. Can be controlled with conventional analgesics, (including NSAIDs if mild, and opioids, if moderate to severe) and in some cases, radiation therapy

    b) Visceral pain: poorly localized; cramping, deep ache, pressure, often referred to distant dermatome sites

        i.   Examples: bowel obstruction, cholecystitis; metastatic tumors in the lung

        ii. Can be controlled with conventional analgesics, and in some cases, antineoplastic treatments

4. Neuropathic pain results from actual injury to nerves rather than stimulation of nerve endings (refer to Table 1 for Pain Terms Associated with Neuropathic Pain States)

    a) Characteristics: sharp, burning, shooting, shock-like, sometimes associated with acyclovir and dysesthesias

    b) Examples: spinal nerve root compression, tumor invasion of nerves, post-herpetic neuralgia, surgical interruption of nerves, central pain syndromes occurring after stroke

    c) Response to conventional analgesics often poor (although this is controversial); but antidepressant, (e.g., nortriptyline) anticonvulsant (e.g., gabapentin, carbamazepine), corticosteroids and non-drug therapies may be beneficial as adjuvant analgesics to the opioids or in some cases as the primary analgesic. Adjuvant analgesics are medications that have a primary indication other than pain; however contain analgesic properties various pain conditions. Adjuvant medications can be used as an add-on to an existing opioid regimen or as a primary therapy for pain where good results are likely to occur[5]

5. Mixed nociceptive and neuropathic pain syndrome

    a) Common in life-threatening illnesses

    b) Thorough assessment is indicated

        i.   Pharmacological therapy is based upon these different pain syndromes

        ii. Occur concomitantly so patients may require agents from more than one category of analgesics (e.g., non-opioids, opioids, and adjuvants)

6. Referred pain is usually a visceral pain referred to skin, bone, and muscle, often distant from the site of origin

   a) Pain from tumor involvement of the pancreas, lower esophagus, stomach or retroperitoneal area may be referred to the back

   b) Gallbladder or liver disease may produce referred pain in the back or right shoulder (suprascapular)

   c) Rectosigmoid involvement may result in pain to sacrum or rectal area

B. Assessment Parameters

1. Site: have patient point on self or diagram, identify and assess all sites as well as sites of radiation; remember, also, the patient may have more than one site of pain; in that case, it would be helpful to number pains to organize assessment, interventions, and evaluations

2. Character: use the patient's *own* words; a careful description will lead to the diagnosis of pain type, and therefore use of appropriate adjuvant analgesics (i.e., sharp, shooting describes neuropathic pain syndromes); refer to the section, "Types of Pain," for additional, in depth descriptions

3. Onset: when did it start? Did (or does) a specific event trigger the pain?

   a) Carefully distinguish between new and pre-existing pain (i.e., arthritis, chronic low back pain syndromes, etc.)

   b) Also assess for breakthrough pain

      i. Transient flares of pain in patients with chronic pain syndromes are referred to as breakthrough pain

      ii. Breakthrough pain can be incidental (e.g., associated with movement), idiopathic (i.e., the cause is not known), or can occur as end-of-dose failure (e.g., the pain recurs prior to the next dose of pain medication)

4. Duration and frequency: how long has the pain persisted? Is it constant or does it come and go (intermittent)?

5. Intensity: *Important note—ratings of pain intensity are the most important piece of pain assessment data to obtain if time is short; pain intensity directly correlates with interference with the patient's quality of life*

   a) Commonly defined on a scale, most frequently 0–10, intensity rating method must be adapted to patient. Record pain intensity "now," at its "worst," at its "least" and on an average. Pain rating scales for cognitively impaired or nonverbal patients are available, but caregivers (be they family or staff in a care facility) can often give valuable information to add to the pain assessment. A change in the patient's behavior, however, is considered the "gold standard"

   b) Indicators of the presence of pain in patients who are unable to respond include the furrowed brow and grimacing

   c) Relief of the furrowing is often seen when pain is relieved; likewise, response to treatment can be considered part of the assessment

   d) Several different pain assessment tools exist, but the basic information is similar. See Figures 1 and 2 for sample tools

Figure 1: Numerical Rating Scale (NRS)

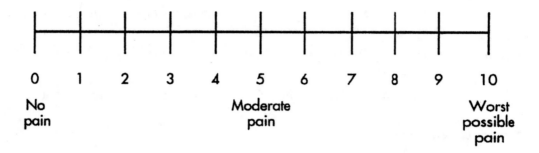

May be duplicated for use in clinical practice. As appears in McCaffery M, Pasero C. Pain: Clinical Manual. St. Louis: MO: Mosby; 1999:67.

Figure 2: Wong-Baker Faces Pain Rating Scale

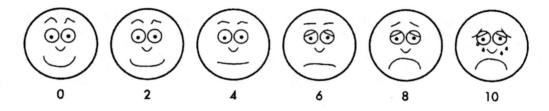

Modified from: Wong DL. Whaley and Wong's Essentials of Pediatric Nursing. 5th ed. St. Louis, MO: Mosby; 1997: 1215–1216.

6. Exacerbating factors: what times, activities, or other circumstances make the pain worse?

7. Associated symptoms: what other symptoms occur before, with or after the pain?

8. Alleviating factors: what makes the pain better? What treatments (including non-pharmacologic interventions) have been successful in the past and what unsuccessful? Include a thorough medication history

9. Medication History: what medications have been ordered? What medications is the patient currently taking? If there is a disparity, examine the underlying reasons (e.g., cost, adverse effects, fears of addiction or tolerance). What medications worked in the past for unrelated pain episodes? What are the patient/family/caregivers' beliefs about opioids?

10. Impact on quality of life: what does the pain mean to the patient and family? How has this pain affected them and their quality of life? Does it keep the patient from doing things he/she wants to do? How much does the patient and the family know about pain? Do they have the expectation that it can be relieved? Are there emotional or spiritual components to the pain? Does unrelieved pain lead to increased fear or anxiety, or to fears that death is imminent?

11. Physical examination: observe the site of the pain, and validate with the patient the pain's location; note skin color, warmth, irritation, integrity and any other unusual findings; utilize other physical assessment techniques, for example, percussion and auscultation, as appropriate; be mindful that persons with chronic or persisent pain often have no changes in vital signs or facial expression

C. Etiology of Pain

1. Cancer Pain Syndromes

   a) Pain associated with direct tumor involvement

      i. Direct tumor involvement accounts for approximately 78% of pain problems among cancer inpatients and 62% among cancer outpatients

      ii. Examples include metastatic bone disease, nerve compression or infiltration, hollow viscus involvement, among others

   b) Pain associated with cancer therapy

      i. Cancer therapy accounts for approximately 19% of pain problems among cancer inpatients and 25% among cancer outpatients

      ii. Examples include any pain that occurs in the course of or as a result of surgery, chemotherapy or radiation therapy (specific examples are mucositis, peripheral neuropathy, phantom pain syndromes, extravasation of vesicant chemotherapy)

   c) Pain unrelated to cancer or cancer therapy

      i. Incident pain accounts for approximately 3% of pain problems among cancer inpatients and 10% of pain problems among cancer outpatients

      ii. Examples include arthritis, osteoporosis, migraine headache, low back pain, fibromyalgia, or any other pain syndromes present among the general population

      iii. Incident pain can also refer to pain that is the result of activity or no movement at all. Breakthrough pain is a type of incident pain

2. Pain syndromes common in the terminal phase of other medical conditions

   a) HIV infection and AIDS

      i. Statistics on the prevalence of pain in AIDS range from 30 to 97%, with an estimate of 50% relating directly to the HIV infection and 30% to the therapy for AIDS

      ii. HIV pain is often categorized in a manner similar to cancer: pain associated with the virus (e.g., direct involvement of the virus in the sensory neurons that transmit pain), pain associated with the treatment (e.g., neuropathy due to antiretroviral drugs) or pain unrelated to HIV or its treatment (e.g., musculoskeletal pains after exercise)

iii. Examples of HIV/AIDS related pain include neuropathies (specifically peripheral neuropathy, acute and chronic polyneuropathy, symmetric distal sensory neuropathy, brachial plexopathy, herpetic neuralgia, cranial neuropathy, and headaches from acute and chronic meningitis), central pain from cerebral abscesses, esophagitis and abdominal pain from infectious gastrointestinal disease, chest pain from pneumocystis pneumonia and generalized myalgias

b) Sickle cell disease

  i. Three or more vascular occlusive episodes are a poor prognostic sign (less than 50% of those patients live beyond age 40). Hydroxyurea may decrease frequency of vaso-occlusive crises

  ii. Pain is severe and acute; focal (bone, joint and muscle) and visceral pain from ischemia and infarction

  iii. There are multiple myths and mistaken beliefs about sickle cell disease and sickle cell pain on the part of patients, their families and the healthcare professions

  iv. Factors related to race, ethnic, and class stereotyping in our culture further complicate this issue and serve as additional impediments to the control of pain in sickle cell disease[6]

c) Multiple sclerosis (MS)

  i. Pain is an issue in 55 to 82% of persons with MS

    (a) Neurological (paroxysmal trigeminal neuralgia, optic neuritis and periorbital pain, extremity pain, including dysesthesia, allodynia and painful electric-shock sensations)

    (b) Musculoskeletal (low back pain and extremity pain) in nature. Refer to Table 2 for definitions of the pain terms associated with neuropathic pain states

d) Cerebral vascular disease

  i. Post stroke pain is a problem in 1–2% of patients

    (a) Often delayed for several years after the stroke; accompanied by decreased temperature sensation; may be superficial or deep; often severe in intensity and accompanied by hyperalgesia and allodynia; may be elicited by emotional episodes and movement

    (b) Another common post-stroke pain syndrome is mechanical shoulder pain unrelated to the central injury

e) Spinal cord injury: central pain may occur from an injury at any level of the spinal cord

D. **Factors that may influence the experience of pain: pain is experienced by the patient *and* family in keeping with the model of "total pain" and includes physical, psychological, social and spiritual effects; when adequate assessment and management of controllable symptoms precede psychological, social and spiritual assessment and intervention, overall outcomes often improve (Remember the lesson in Maslow's Hierarchy of needs); common effects of pain include**

1. Physical effects: decreased functional ability, including ability to walk and perform other basic ADLs, decreased strength and endurance, nausea, anorexia, insomnia and impaired immune response

2. Psychosocial effects: alteration in social and close relationships, isolation, inability to work; loss of self-esteem, self-worth; increased caregiver burden, further disruption of important social supports for both patient and family

3. Emotional effects: diminished leisure, increased fear and anxiety, depression, hopelessness, despair, loss of control; if pain uncontrolled, consideration of suicide or physician assisted suicide

4. Spiritual issues: increased suffering, re-evaluation and perhaps doubt regarding past religious foundations and beliefs; questioning the meaning of suffering

5. Financial effects: inability to work and earn income, loss of caregiver income, issues of workplace discrimination, and having to apply for governmental assistance leading to decreased income and loss of health insurance coverage

6. Cultural issues: ethnic minority, female, and elderly persons often receive less than optimal pain management in all settings[7]

   a) Consider the patient's family of origin, their manner of expressing pain, and how suffering is valued

   b) Perceptions of pain, end of life, afterlife, bereavement and other aspects of palliative care vary widely by ethnicity and within ethnicities

   c) Be careful of "stereotyping," and do everything possible to learn about the patient and family's unique situation

   d) Specific aspects of culture to assess when caring for patients in pain include ethnic identity, gender, age, differing abilities, sexual orientation, religion and spirituality, financial status, place of residency, employment and educational level

III. Pharmacologic Intervention[1]

A. Types of Pharmacologic Interventions

1. Drug actions and side effects

   a) Aspirin-like drugs (salicylates, and non-salicylates [NSAIDs])

      i. Actions: analgesic, antipyretic, anti-inflammatory, antithrombotic

      ii. Adverse effects

---

[1] Thanks to June L. Dahl, PhD, Professor of Pharmacology at the University of Wisconsin-Madison Medical School for her assistance with this section.

    (a)   GI distress; no relation between symptoms and seriousness of GI effects; concomitant administration of misoprostol (Cytotec®) or a proton pump inhibitor (e.g., omeprazole [Prilosec®]) can prevent gastropathy

    (b)   Renal insufficiency: elderly and dehydrated are at increased risk

    (c)   Inhibiting of platelet aggregation

    (d)   Hypersensitivity reactions (not allergic reactions); symptoms include urticaria, bronchospasm, severe rhinitis, and shock

        (i)   Adverse effects are often labeled by patients/caregivers as "allergies" (e.g., nausea and vomiting)

        (ii)   These are not absolute contraindications to using the drug

    (e)   CNS effects: dizziness, tinnitus, decreased hearing, headache

    iii.   Dose escalation is limited by analgesic ceiling

b)   Acetaminophen

    i.   Actions: analgesic, antipyretic, *not anti-inflammatory*

    ii.   Adverse effects: far fewer than with NSAIDs; hepatotoxic in large doses; ceiling is 4 grams a day, lower in alcoholic patients, AIDS patients, patients with liver metastasis or those with active liver disease. Dose escalation is limited by analgesic ceiling—consider quantity of acetaminophen in combination medications (refer to Table 1)

c)   Opioid medications

    i.   Pure agonists (morphine is prototype, others include fentanyl, hydrocodone, hydromorphone, methadone, oxycodone)

    ii.   Mixed agonist-antagonists (pentazocine (Talwin®), butorphanol (Stadol®), nalbuphine (Nubain®); *not recommended for the treatment of cancer pain due to analgesic ceiling, psychotomimetic affect, precipitation of withdrawal when given to patients on opioids*

    iii.   Action: bind to receptors in the brain, spinal cord and in periphery

    iv.   Side effects of opioids

        (a)   Tolerance develops in days to weeks[2,3] to the sedative, emetic and respiratory depressant effects of opioids; however it does not develop to constipation

        (b)   Sedation, sometimes, but rarely confusion

        (c)   Dizziness, dysphoria

        (d)   Nausea

        (e)   Constipation—tolerance <u>does not</u> develop—*must be prevented and treated aggressively*

        (f)   Itching and urticaria

(g) Respiratory depression

   (i) Feared and misunderstood

   (ii) Clinically significant respiratory depression is extremely rare when patients in severe pain receive opioids, especially in patients who are currently receiving opioids and when doses are titrated upward in appropriate steps; there are not good data to support the prevalence of respiratory depression due to opioids, however, there is general agreement that patients who are at risk are those who are opioid naïve and concomitantly taking other sedating drugs

   (iii) Respiratory rate alone is not an indicator of respiratory depression; some patients may have a respiratory rate of 7, while alert and well perfused; other factors that must be considered are the level of sedation, the depth of respiration, and the adequacy of perfusion of oxygen in the tissues as determined by examining nail beds for changes in color, or obtaining an oxygen saturation level or pulse oximmetry

v. Some other drug adverse effects include

  (a) Meperidine (Demerol®)

   (i) Converted to a long-lived excitatory metabolite (normeperidine) causing shaky feelings, tremors/twitches, and myoclonus/grand mal seizures; should not be used in cancer pain management, can cause hallucinations and is contraindicated for elders

   (ii) Poor oral bioavailability

  (b) Propoxyphene, the opioid in Darvon® and Darvocet® although widely prescribed

   (i) Is an ineffective analgesic

   (ii) Has a long-lived metabolite toxic to the central nervous system and cardiovascular system

   (iii) Is combined with a large amount of acetaminophen. Therefore, it is not recommended for long-term use or use in the elderly. No more than 4 gms of acetaminophen should be given in 24 hours due to its toxic effect on the liver

  (c) Morphine

   (i) Active metabolites (morphine 3- glucuronide[M3G], morphine 6-glucuronide[M6G]), excreted by the kidneys will be retained by elderly patients and by those with diminished renal function; has strong analgesic and respiratory depressant properties; M3G may produce central nervous system hyper-excitability and possibly myoclonus, while elevated M6G levels appear to cause sedation

   (ii) Small amounts of hydration (IV fluids at 30-50cc/hr) helps to clear it through the kidneys

   (iii) Hydromorphone may be a safer choice for the elderly or those with diminished renal function

    vi.   Most opioids do not have a ceiling dose—so able to titrate to effect. Check with your pharmacist for those that have a ceiling dose. All mixed agonist/antagonists do have dosage ceilings and thus cannot be titrated to effect

        (a)   Opioids that are administered in combination with another medication such as acetaminophen or aspirin, do have dose limitations due to the acetaminophen or aspirin

    vii.   Delivery routes

        (a)   Oral: most preferred for comfort, convenience, and cost effectiveness; many forms available, immediate release tablets, sustained release tablets, liquids; Oralet® (fentanyl) is available as well. Sublingual is same as oral route

        (b)   Rectal: useful for patients who are NPO or have nausea and vomiting; contraindicated with anal lesions, diarrhea, constipation, or leukopenia; varying comfort levels with family caregivers and some cultures

        (c)   Subcutaneous or intravenous infusion: rarely required, but useful for pain requiring rapid titration of medication; while subcutaneous infusion is useful in most cases, impaired circulation or the presence of fibrosis can compromise absorption; used extensively at home for patients who are obstructed or who can no longer swallow and have severe pain. Can be managed within home setting; especially useful if parenteral route required and reliable or intravenous access not possible. Expense of home parenteral infusions to hospice programs are a barrier to use

        (d)   Intramuscular injections should be avoided, injections are painful, unnecessary and absorption is not reliable

        (e)   Transmucosal: easily accessible route, provides rapid onset of action and is much faster if used with lipophilic drugs such as fentanyl

        (f)   Transdermal (e.g., fentanyl) for patients with stable pain (not good for rapid titration of medication); reservoir in subcutaneous tissue, delayed onset of action (12–24 hours), so patient must have an immediate release medication during the first several hours after the fentanyl patch is applied, some patients require a patch change every 48 hours; should not be given to opioid naïve patients

        (g)   Spinal: via indwelling catheters into the epidural or intrathecal space; an implantable pump should be used in only carefully selected patients after appropriate consultation; cost, care issues, and potential adverse effects should also be carefully weighed however can dramatically improve some patients quality of life especially with severe pain in lower extremities

d) Adjuvant analgesics: drugs that have a primary indication other than pain (e.g., antidepressant or anticonvulsant) but are also analgesic for some painful conditions

    i. For treatment of neuropathic pain

       (a) Tricyclic antidepressants

         (i) Desipramine and nortriptyline recommended over amitriptyline, which has more anticholinergic effects (causing cardiovascular changes, dry mouth, constipation)

         (ii) Serotonin selective reuptake inhibitors (SSRIs) have not been well studied in neuropathic pain and may seem to have limited analgesic effect

         (iii) Guidelines for monitoring

            (a) These drugs may cause sedation and enhance sleep

            (b) Response may be delayed by 3–7 days

            (c) Monitor adverse effects

            (d) Adverse effects: sedation, orthostatic hypotension, anticholinergic side effects (including urinary retention), cardiac effects

       (b) Anticonvulsants

         (i) Most useful for lancinating, paroxysmal pain and pain that does not respond to antidepressant therapy; dose as with seizures; most experience has been with carbamazepine

         (ii) Gabapentin (300–1800 mg TID); carbamazepine (100–800 mg BID or QID); phenytoin (100–200 mg TID); valproic acid (200–400 mg BID or TID); clonazepam (0.25–.5 mg TID); (all doses are po)

         (iii) Guidelines for monitoring

            (a) Watch for side effects

            (b) Monitor carbamazepine, phenytoin and valproic acid serum levels for signs of toxicity

         (iv) Major adverse effects

            (a) Gabapentin: sedation, side effects generally less than with others (has less bone marrow suppression—drug of choice for patients on chemotherapy); costly

            (b) Carbamazepine: bone marrow suppression, vertigo, confusion, sedation

            (c) Phenytoin: ataxia, rash, hepatotoxicity

            (d) Valproic acid: nausea, vomiting, sedation, ataxia, tremor, thrombocytopenia, neutropenia, hepatotoxicity

            (e) Clonazepam: sedation, physical dependence

    (c)   Local anesthetics

        (i)   Useful in refractory neuropathic pain

        (ii)   Lidocaine, given IV (more likely to be offered outside hospice program); tocainide (Tonocard®) and mexiletine (Mexiletine®), given orally. Mexiletine must be titrated very slowly and serum levels monitored

        (iii)   Adverse effects include dizziness, lightheadedness, lowered blood pressure, sensory disturbances and tremor, seizures at high doses, nausea and vomiting

        (iv)   Lidocaine 5% is also available in a patch for topical relief of post-herpetic neuropathy, post-thoracotomy pain and other pain syndromes

            (a)   The patches should be placed over intact skin only

            (b)   Up to three patches can be used to cover the painful area and are left in place for 12 hours, with 12 hours off

            (c)   Adverse effects are uncommon and include pain with removal of the patch

            (d)   Patients with sensitivity to touch (also called allodynia) often report relief

    (d)   Baclofen (muscle relaxant): used to treat a variety of neuropathic pain problems

    ii.   Corticosteroids: used in metastatic bone pain (triple effect of pain control, mood elevation and increased appetite)

    iii.   Topical capsaicin: may be used for diabetic neuropathy, post-herpetic neuralgia, arthritis and Kaposi's Sarcoma lesions though there are newer medications that are more effective and do not cause irritation and pain when applied

    iv.   Other medications used to treat side effects of opioids e.g., psychostimulants, phenothiazines, benzodiazepines (muscle spasms)

B.   **Non-pharmacologic interventions can be used concurrently with pharmacological and other modalities to relieve pain and can often be taught to patients and/or family members; there are some who believe that medications should never be given without the addition of <u>some</u> non-pharmacologic intervention. However, the use of non-pharmacologic interventions should <u>never</u> preclude appropriate use of medications, including opioids. The most common non-pharmacologic interventions are listed below**

    1.   Physical modalities

        a)   Consider physical therapy (PT) and occupational therapy (OT) consults (especially in the inpatient palliative care setting)

        b)   Cutaneous stimulation (heat, cold)

        c)   Exercise (with limitations based on physical condition)

d) Transcutaneous nerve stimulation (efficacy controversial may be useful in patients with mild pain); acupuncture

e) Massage; healing touch; therapeutic touch

2. Psychosocial and spiritual interventions (helpful in maintaining control in uncertain, dependent and anxiety-provoking situations)

a) Relaxation and guided imagery

b) Distraction

c) Music

d) Reframing

e) Patient/family education

f) Hypnosis

g) Counseling

h) Prayer

i) Spiritual reflection or meditation

3. Other

a) Biofeedback

b) Aromatherapy

4. Palliative radiation therapy

a) May be used to relieve symptoms of patients with advanced disease, (e.g., pain, bleeding), compression of vital organ systems, (e.g., the brain, ulcerating skin lesions) and metastasis to weight bearing bones susceptible to fracture

b) Radiation therapy is the treatment of choice for spinal cord compression, bone pain and is frequently used in superior vena cava syndrome and symptomatic brain metastases

c) While external beam radiation is the modality commonly used for palliative radiation therapy, Strontium-89 and Samarium Sm-153 are intravenous radionucleotides that emits beta radiation at the bony metastatic site, is sometimes used to treat areas of painful skeletal metastasis; newer radionucleotides are currently under study that may not produce the painful flair that occurs when Strontium-89 is given

5. Palliative chemotherapy: may improve or enhance comfort when neither cure nor control is possible

a) Antineoplastic therapy may produce tumor shrinkage, relief of pressure on nerves, lymphatics, and blood vessels and reduction in organ obstruction, thus relieving pain

b) Bisphosphonates are useful in treating pain related to multiple myeloma and metastatic bone disease[2]

IV. Pain during the Final Days of Life

A. Pain Assessment

1. Patients may become nonverbal in the final days of life

   a) A furrowed brow may indicate pain

   b) Guarding and vocalization during turning or dressing changes may suggest pain

   c) A therapeutic trial of an opioid should be strongly considered to determine if these behaviors change with the use of an analgesic

2. If the patient had pain prior to becoming unresponsive, assume pain is still present

B. Pharmacologic Management

1. As organ system dysfunction increases, particularly renal clearance, drugs or their metabolites are cleared from the body less efficiently and sedation may increase

   a) Therefore, a therapeutic trial of opioid dose reduction may be indicated if sedation is not a desired effect

   b) In some cases, patients may become more alert and responsive

   c) If any signs of pain return, the dose should be returned to its previous level

2. Rapid discontinuation of opioids, benzodiazepines or other agents can result in the abstinence syndrome; whenever possible, gradual reduction in dose of these drugs is indicated

3. Sedation at the end of life is an option for patients with intractable pain and suffering[2]

   a) There are numerous combinations of medications that are used to accomplish sedation

      i. Opioids

      ii. Barbiturates

      iii. Neuroleptics

      iv. Benzodiazepines

   b) Therapy is based on obtaining initial relief of symptoms followed by ongoing sedation to maintain the effect

   c) Parenteral ketamine, given either as a continuous infusion or as bolus doses, may also be used to accomplish sedation at the end of life

C. Non-pharmacologic management should continue

V.   Summary of Principles of Pain Management

A.   Pain assessment data is documented so the pain etiology or syndrome can be identified and appropriately treated

B.   The oral route is used whenever possible

1.   If the patient is unable to take oral medications, buccal, sublingual, rectal, and transdermal routes are considered before parenteral routes

2.   IM route is avoided

3.   IV and subcutaneous route can be used for any patient that cannot tolerate above choices under oral route or when pain is rapidly escalating and severe. Subcutaneous route is a useful alternative in the home setting when reliable IV access is not possible

C.   Constant pain calls for treatment with an around-the-clock scheduled long acting opioid and a short acting medication for breakthrough pain

1.   Only one long-acting opioid is ordered for constant pain

2.   Doses of opioids are increased commensurate with the patient's report of pain

3.   Equianalgesic conversions are used when changing medications and/or routes

4.   Adjuvant medications are used for neuropathic pain, some visceral pain states, and bone pain

D.   Breakthrough pain

1.   Only one analgesic is ordered for breakthrough pain. Ideally the same drug should be used for breakthrough pain as long acting if available (e.g., long acting MS Contin® and MSIR® for breakthrough pain)

2.   A higher dosage of breakthrough, or rescue medication, is sometimes necessary if the frequency of breakthrough pain and/or intensity are at higher levels; this dose will be determined by the physician with the assistance of the registered nurse and pharmacist

3.   Patients and families need to be educated about taking the medication when the pain is first perceived—not when it has become severe or unbearable

E.   Non-pharmacologic approaches are always a part of any pain management plan

F.   An appropriate preventative bowel regimen is ordered with a stimulant laxative and stool softener to correct the effects of the opioid. (see Chapter V)

VI. **Evaluation—pain management is predicated by ongoing assessment of treatment efficacy and control of treatment side effects**

    A. **Evaluation of interventions is a basic nursing function and completes the nursing process; all nursing personnel contribute in this function**

    B. **Nursing evaluation should be accomplished in a timely manner, in accordance with expected pharmacologic peak action or when the non-pharmacologic intervention is completed**

    C. **At each nursing contact with a patient assess for**

        1. Pain intensity, type, duration, etc.

        2. Medication side effects, interactions or complications

        3. Patient's satisfaction with method of pain relief

    D. **In the inpatient setting**

        1. Pain assessment every shift or more frequently as indicated

        2. Patient/family teaching and reinforcement of pain management

        3. Monitor fluid intake, activity tolerance and bowel status daily and document

    E. **Evaluate efficacy of pain relief interventions**

        1. At appropriate intervals after any change in medication, dosage, route of administration, etc.

        2. At each nursing contact with a patient

Table 1: Combination Products

Opioid	Proprietary Name and Combination Drugs[a]
Hydrocodone	Vicodin® (5mg + 500mg acetaminophen) Vicodin ES® (7.5mg + 750mg acetaminophen) Lorcet-10® (10mg + 650mg acetaminophen) Lortab® Vicodin HP® (10mg + 660mg acetaminophen) Norco® (10mg + 325mg acetaminophen) Anexsia® (5mg + 500mg acetaminophen) Zydone® (5mg + 400mg acetaminophen)
Oxycodone	Percodan® (5mg + 325mg ASA) Percocet® (5mg + 325mg acetaminophen) Tylox® (5mg + 500mg acetaminophen) Roxicet® (5mg + 325mg acetaminophen)
Codeine	Tylenol #2® (15mg + 325mg acetaminophen) Tylenol #3® (30mg + 325mg acetaminophen) Tylenol #4® (60mg + 325mg acetaminophen)
Propoxyphene[b]	Darvon® (65mg) Darvocet N®® (100mg + 650mg acetaminophen) Darvon Compound® (65mg + 325mg ASA + caffeine) Darvon-N® or Darvon® with ASA (65mg + 325mg ASA)

[a]Twenty-four hour dose of acetaminophen should not exceed 4 grams for adults

[b]WARNING: Long-lived metabolite that is toxic to the central nervous system and cardiovascular system, not recommended for long-term use and use in the elderly.

Table 2: Pain Terms Associated with Neuropathic Pain States

Modified from the International Association for the Study of Pain; McCaffery and Pasero.

Term	Definition	
Allodynia	Pain due to a stimulus, which does not normally provoke pain	
Dysesthesia	An unpleasant abnormal sensation, whether spontaneous or evoked	
Hyperalgesia	A painful syndrome characterized by an abnormally painful reaction to a normally non-painful stimulus, such as touch. (Sometimes referred hyperpathia)	
Paresthesia	An abnormal anesthetic sensation (often described as a painful numbness)	
Neuralgia	Pain in the distribution of a nerve or nerves	
Neuropathic pain	Pain initiated or caused by a primary lesion or dysfunction in the nervous system	
	Peripheral neuropathic pain	Pain initiated or caused by a primary lesion or dysfunction in the peripheral nervous system (e.g., post-herpetic neuropathy).
	Central pain	Pain initiated or caused by a primary lesion or dysfunction in the central nervous system. (e.g., post-thalamic pain syndrome occurring after stroke)

CITED REFERENCES

1. McCaffery M, Pasero C. *Pain: Clinical Manual.* St. Louis, MO: Mosby; 1999.

2. Paice JA, Fine P. Pain at the end of life. In: Ferrell B, Coyle N, eds. *Textbook of Palliative Nursing.* New York, NY: Oxford University Press; 2001:76–90.

3. Coyle N, Layman-Goldstein M. Pain assessment and management in palliative care. In: Matzo ML, Sherman DW, eds. *Palliative Care Nursing: Quality Care to the End of Life.* New York, NY: Springer Publishing; 2001:362–468.

4. World Health Organization. Cancer: Palliative Care. Available at http://www.who.int/cancer/palliative/en/. Accessed March 1, 2005.

5. Portenoy R. Adjuvant analgesics in pain management. In: Doyle D, Hanks G, MacDonald N, eds. Oxford Textbook of Palliative Medicine. 2nd ed. New York, NY: Oxford University Press; 1998:361–362.

6. Benjamin LJ, Dampler CD, Jacox A, et al. *Guidelines for the Management of Acute and Chronic Pain in Sickle-Cell Disease.* Skokie, IL: American Pain Society; 1999.

7. Cleelan C, et al. Pain and its treatment in outpatients with metastatic cancer. *New England Journal of Medicine,* 1994;330:592–596.

ADDITIONAL REFERENCES AND RESOURCES

Griffie, J., Muchka, S., & Weissman, D.E. (2000). *Nursing Staff Education Resource Manual: Pain Management 101.* Milwaukee, WI: Palliative Care Program, Medical College of Wisconsin. Available from: www.mcw.edu/palmed/.

Gordon DB, Dahl JL, Stevenson KK. *Building an Institutional Commitment to Pain Management: The Wisconsin Resource Manual.* 2nd ed. Madison, WI: University of Wisconsin-Madison Board of Regents; 2000.

Kovach C, Griffie J, Muchka S, Noonan P, Weissman DE. Nurses' perceptions of pain assessment and treatment in cognitively impaired elderly. *Clinical Nurse Specialist.* 2000;14:215–220.

Panke JT. Difficulties in managing pain at the end of life. *Journal of Hospice and Palliative Nursing.* 2002:5(2):83–90.

Shaver WA. Suffering and the role of abandonment of self. *Journal of Hospice and Palliative Nursing.* 2002:4(1):46–53.

SUPPORT Study Principle Investigators. A controlled trial to improve care for seriously ill hospitalized patients: a study to understand prognoses and preferences for outcomes and risks of treatments (SUPPORT). *Journal of the American Medical Association.* 1995;274:1591–1598.

Weissman DE, Griffie J, Muchka S, Matson S. Building an institutional commitment to pain management in long term care facilities. *Journal of Pain and Symptom Management.* 2000;20:35–43.

Wrede-Seaman L. *Symptom Management Algorithms: A Handbook for Palliative Care.* 2nd ed. Yakima, WA: Intellicard; 1999.

Zerwekh J, Riddell S, Richard J. Fearing to comfort: a grounded theory of constraints to opioid use in hospice. *Journal of Hospice and Palliative Nursing.* 2002:4(2):83–90.

CHAPTER V

SYMPTOM MANAGEMENT

Roger Strong, APRN, BC-PCM

Adapted from: Collins CA, Wilson MA. Symptom Management.
In: Volker BG, Watson AC, eds. *Core Curriculum for the Generalist Hospice and Palliative Nurse.*
Dubuque, IA: Kendall/Hunt Publishing Company; 2002: 89–154.

I. **Principles**

    A. **The nursing process (using assessment, diagnosis, planning, for symptom management and care at the end of life)**

    B. **Care at the end of life is multidimensional with emphasis on quality-of-life as the patient and family define it, with respect for, support and education of patient and family**

    C. **Understanding of expectations, goals of treatment, end-of-life goals. Issues must be clarified with patient and family, taking into account the patient's position on the disease trajectory**

    D. **The interdisciplinary team (IDT) is the framework for palliative care and hospice**

    E. **The patient and family are the unit of care in palliative care and hospice and are included in the assessment, planning, decision-making and evaluation of interventions**

        1. Options and expected or possible outcomes are discussed with patient and family to inform their decision making; the IDT is responsible for giving them information regarding the benefits and the burdens of any treatment that is proposed

        2. Patients and families require time, opportunity for clarification and review in anticipation of making decisions

    F. **The end of life can be a time of growth, reconciliation, peace, joy and hope for patients and families; appropriate symptom management can facilitate this process by maximizing patient comfort**

G. **Authors' note: Patients may experience a variety of symptoms. Those covered in this chapter are some of the most often experienced by individuals with life-threatening illness**

II. Alteration in Skin and Mucous Membranes

A. **Definition: disruption in the integrity of the skin or oral mucous membrane**

B. **Possible Etiologies**

1. Skin integrity

   a) Pressure ulcers

      i. Pressure to the skin, causing a decrease in blood flow and eventual cell death

      ii. Shearing forces, in which two surfaces slide in opposite but parallel directions (e.g., a patient slides down in bed and bone and skin are displaced from one another)

      iii. Friction, in which two surfaces move across one another (e.g., patient is dragged across bed sheets)

      iv. Moisture (especially feces and urine)

      v. Obesity

      vi. Malnutrition

      vii. Immobility

      viii. Impaired circulation due to peripheral vascular disease, diabetes or cancer infiltration through skin

   b) Fistulas

   c) Tumor necrosis

2. Alteration of oral mucous membranes

   a) Dry mouth (xerostomia)

      i. Candidiasis

      ii. Drugs (anticholinergics, antihistamines, phenothiazines)

      iii. Radiation and chemotherapy

      iv. Dehydration

      v. Mucositis

      vi. Mouth breathing

      vii. Metabolic disorders (hypercalcemia, hyperglycemia)

   b) Candidiasis

      i. Radiation and chemotherapy

      ii. Drugs (antibiotics, corticosteroids)

      c)   Herpes simplex virus

      d)   Mucositis caused by radiation or chemotherapy

3.   Pruritus: uncomfortable itching of the skin

      a)   Dry, flaky skin

      b)   Wet, macerated skin

      c)   Contact dermatitis caused by ointments or creams

      d)   Infestations caused by scabies, lice, fleas

      e)   Drugs (antibiotics, morphine, phenothiazines)

      f)   Systemic disease (renal failure, hepatobiliary disease, infiltration of tumors into subcutaneous tissue)

      g)   Fungal infections

C.   Assess For

1.   Skin integrity

      a)   Inspect skin each time patient changes position

      b)   If pressure ulcer, grade wound according to stage[1]

          i.   Stage I: Non-blanchable erythema of intact skin, the heralding lesion of skin ulceration

             (a)   In individuals with dark skin, discoloration of the skin, warmth, edema, induration or hardness also may be indicators

             (b)   Skin changes may be difficult to discern in some persons of color and the patient's report of pain may be the only cue to closely examine at-risk areas; be mindful of baseline skin color and monitor skin frequently for skin color change

         ii.   Stage II: Partial thickness skin loss involving epidermis, dermis, or both. The ulcer is superficial and presents clinically as an abrasion, blister or shallow crater

         iii.   Stage III: Full thickness skin loss involving damage to or necrosis of subcutaneous tissue that may extend down to, but not through, underlying fascia. The ulcer presents clinically as a deep crater with or without undermining of adjacent tissue

         iv.   Stage IV: Full thickness skin loss with extensive destruction, tissue necrosis, or damage to muscle, bone, or supporting structures; undermining and sinus tracts also may be associated with Stage IV pressure ulcers

      c)   Wound location

      d)   Wound appearance

          i.   Size, length, width, depth, undermining

          ii.   Presence of drainage (serous, serosanguineous, sanguineous, purulent) and amount

          iii.   Tissue type (i.e., granulating or eschar)

          iv.   Appearance of surrounding skin (redness, maceration, etc.)

      e)   Is wound painful?

      f)   If wound is due to tumor necrosis, does the location present a potential for serious complications (i.e., potential for hemorrhage or obstruction of blood flow due to the tumor located next to blood vessels)?

      g)   Is the wound malodorous or fungating?

      h)   A nutritional assessment is important, as malnutrition can impede proper wound healing and also cause pressure ulcer formation

2.   Alteration in Oral Mucous Membranes

      a)   Patient history of mouth dryness or sore mouth

      b)   Review of medications which may cause oral membrane alterations (i.e., antibiotics, chemotherapy drugs such as IV 5-Fluouracil, anticholinergics)

      c)   Examination of internal and external oral mucosa

          i.   Dry, cracked lips

          ii.   Sores or white patches on buccal membranes, oropharynx or tongue

          iii.   Bleeding of gums, lips or tongue

      d)   Patient's current oral hygiene regimen

      e)   Patient and family knowledge of etiology and management of altered oral mucous membranes

3.   Pruritus

      a)   History of itching (including when, how long, what is tolerable)

      b)   Assessment of skin

          i.   Presence of rashes or lesions

          ii.   Presence of abrasions from frequent scratching

          iii.   Overall skin integrity

      c)   Review plan of care for medications that may cause pruritus

D. Diagnoses

1. Impaired skin integrity, oral, related to dry mouth, oral lesions, infection

2. Impaired skin integrity related to immobility and pressure over bony prominences

3. Impaired skin integrity related to tumor necrosis or fistula

4. Pain related to altered skin or oral mucous membranes or pruritus

5. Body image disturbance related to malodorous or unsightly wounds

6. Patient/family knowledge deficit related to etiology and management of wounds, altered oral mucous membranes, or pruritus

E. Planning and Intervention

1. Wound management

   a) Relieve pressure

      i. Turn at least every two hours

      ii Place patient on pressure relief and pressure reduction support surfaces

   b) Reduce friction and shearing forces

      i. Teach family proper techniques for moving patient in bed; physical therapy referral may be indicated

      ii. Use transparent dressings or elbow and knee protectors

   c) Consult team dietitian for nutritional assessment and plan of care

   d) Consult enterostomal therapy (ET) nurse for wound management plan, if appropriate

   e) Consult Agency for Healthcare Research and Quality (AHRQ) (formerly AHCPR) guidelines for skin and wound care

   f) Wounds should be cleansed and irrigated with normal saline prior to being dressed

      i. Dressing selection

         (a) The following should be considered when selecting a dressing[1]

            (i) Moist wound bed

            (ii) Dry surrounding skin

            (iii) Exudate control

            (iv) Caregiver time

         (b) If wounds are malodorous, special dressings are required to assist with odor control

            (i) Metronidazole tablets crushed and sprinkled into the malodorous wound will help minimize infection and odor

         (c) Table 1 lists different types of dressings and the types of wounds for which they are appropriate

ii.   Assure adequate pain control prior to changing dressings; utilize topical pain relievers as appropriate for ongoing pain (i.e., topical lidocaine, cold packs)

2.   Alteration in oral mucous membranes

a)   Xerostomia

i.   Stimulate salivation

(a)   Peppermint water

(b)   Gum, mints, hard candy (preferably sugar free to protect teeth)

(c)   Ice chips or frequent sips of water

(d)   Pilocarpine 2.5 mg po tid, titrate to 10 mg po tid; do not use in patients with severe COPD or bowel obstruction[2]

b)   Utilize saliva substitutes

i.   Ice chips or frequent sips of water

ii.   Artificial saliva

c)   Treat dehydration

i.   Ice chips or frequent sips of water

ii.   Offer fluids throughout the day, especially with meals

iii.   Humidify the room

iv.   Place spray bottle and moistened oral swabs close to patient (avoid lemon-glycerin swabs)

d)   Review medications, and alter regimen if appropriate

3.   Sore mouth due to oral Candida, herpetic lesions, mucositis or stomatitis

a)   For Candida, nystatin swish and swallow or fluconazole tablets or suspension

b)   Around-the-clock mouth care at least every two to four hours with moistened oral swabs and saline mouth rinse, if patient is able; be sure to apply water-soluble lubricant to lips

c)   1:4 hydrogen peroxide and water rinse for mucous or hard debris in mouth[3]

d)   Do not serve hot or overly spicy foods; serve softened and moist foods rather than dry

e)   Several oral medications and medicated mouthwash cocktails are available for mouth pain and lesions. Some examples are

i.   Topical morphine

ii.   Viscous lidocaine

iii.   Cocktail of Milk of Magnesia, diphenhydrAMINE, and viscous lidocaine

iv.   Sucralfate slurry

4. Pruritus Interventions

    a) Non-pharmacologic measures

        i. Avoid skin irritants that may cause dryness or additional moisture[4]

           (a) Alcohol

           (b) Tight or heavy clothing

           (c) Frequent bathing with harsh soaps and hot water

        ii. Avoid heat, maintain cool room temperatures; keep the patient cool to avoid sweating, and frequently cleanse the skin with neutral pH cleansers and tepid water

        iii. Cool starch baths

        iv. Cold compresses can decrease itching; make sure to assess skin frequently during application, and do not apply if patient's peripheral vascular system is compromised

        v. Apply lubricating ointments or creams to skin (i.e., lanolin, Udder Cream®) to avoid excessive drying

        vi. Avoid alcohol, foods/drinks containing caffeine, theophylline

    b) Pharmacologic Measures

        i. Antihistamines such as hydroxyzine and diphenhydrAMINE

        ii. Topical corticosteroids can be used for acute localized itching, but should be avoided for chronic pruritis[4]

        iii. Ondansetron and cholestyramine have been used in cholestatic, uremic, and opioid-induced pruritis[4]

        iv. Antifungal creams for pruritus related to Candida

        v. Transcutaneous electrical nerve stimulation (TENS) units may be helpful in localized pruritis[3,4]

F. Patient/Family Education

1. Wounds

    a) Demonstrate correct positioning to maximize pressure relief. Explain importance of changing patient's position every two hours, when appropriate, even if the patient is sitting in a chair

    b) Demonstrate proper technique in moving patient up in bed to reduce friction and shearing force

    c) Demonstrate correct procedures for cleansing and dressing wounds

    d) Explain possible complications with tumor necrotic wounds; prepare family for bleeding or airway concerns and management

    e) Explain management of ostomy bags if fistula present

2.   Altered oral mucous membranes

    a)   Demonstrate proper technique for oral care; explain importance of frequent oral care

    b)   Explain medication usage and potential side effects

    c)   Introduce non-pharmacologic methods for preventing and relieving dry and sore oral mucous membranes

3.   Pruritus

    a)   Explain etiology of pruritus

    b)   Explain ways of preventing pruritus (keep skin clean and dry, avoid soaps, etc.)

    c)   Explain actions of medications and potential side effects

    d)   Introduce non-pharmacologic methods for preventing and relieving pruritus (See Section E, 4 a) above)

G.   Evaluate

1.   Wounds

    a)   Response of patient/family to teaching

    b)   Effectiveness of interventions (i.e., is wound healing?)

    c)   Need for change in plan (i.e., change in dressing, referral to ET nurse)

    d)   Patient/family understanding of treatment and prevention of further alteration of skin integrity

2.   Altered oral mucous membranes and pruritus

    a)   Response to interventions and patient/family teaching

    b)   Effectiveness of interventions: are patient/family satisfied with outcome?

    c)   Medication effects and side effects

    d)   Patient/family understanding of treatment and prevention of further alteration

H.   Revise plan according to findings from ongoing evaluations, changes in patient status or family needs

Table 1: Indications and Uses for Dressings

Type of Dressing	Indications and Uses
Semipermeable film	Protects very early damage from shear forces. Prevents bacterial contamination. Maintains humidity in shallow ulcers, producing ideal conditions for granulation and healing. Provides immediate pain relief. Best applied when there is no exudation from the wound.
Hydrocolloids	For low-exudate wounds. Maintains moist environment. Fluidizes to produce a gel useful for debridement. Provides environment for granulation. Available as a paste to fill wound cavities.
Alginates	For heavy exudates; controls secretion and bacterial contamination by absorption and formation of hydrophilic gel.
Hydrogels/xerogel	For debridement in the presence of slough and infection: rehydrates eschar and makes it easier to remove.
Enzymatic	For eschar and necrotic tissue; loosens necrotic tissue by liquefaction, thereby aiding in its removal. (Protect edges of wound with zinc paste and apply to eschar under an occlusive dressing.)
Polysaccharide dextranomer	For exudative, infected wounds; on contact with wound exudates the beads absorb fluid and swell, forming a gel; bacteria and dead cells are drawn away from the wound. Applied every 24 hours until wound is clean and granulation tissue is developing.
Charcoal	Malodorous infected pressure sores: adsorbs bacteria, cellular debris, toxins, and odors.

Reprinted from *Handbook of Palliative Care in Cancer,* 2nd ed., A. Waller and N. L. Caroline, p. 97, Copyright 2000 with permission from Elsevier.

III. Altered Mental Status: Confusion, Delirium, Terminal Restlessness, Agitation

A. Confusion/Delirium/Agitation

1. Definitions

    a) Confusion

        i. Clouding of consciousness, memory impairment

        ii. Change in cognition/impaired cognitive function, impaired perceptions and emotional disturbances

        iii. May be accompanied by reduced level of consciousness, disorientation and misperceptions

    b) Delirium

        i. Exaggerated emotions or memories with aggression, paranoia or terror displayed

        ii. Disturbance of consciousness with reduced ability to focus

        iii. Disturbance develops over a short period of time (hours or days) and tends to fluctuate over the course of the day

    c) Agitation

        i. Can occur at any time during a disease process and is an objective result of confusion or delirium

        ii. A group of symptoms that may include physically and/or verbally aggressive behaviors, hiding or hoarding behaviors and physically non-aggressive behaviors, i.e., pacing, inappropriate dressing/undressing, repetitive actions[5]

2. Potential Etiologies

    a) Medications: opioids, phenothiazines, benzodiazepines, anticholinergics, beta-blockers, diuretics, dopaminergics, steroids, atropine, phenytoin, H_2 antagonists, digoxin only when toxic

    b) Unrelieved pain, discomfort or other unrelieved symptoms

    c) Full bladder or bowel

    d) Infection (UTI, lung, septicemia)

    e) Brain tumor, primary or metastatic

    f) Cardiac or respiratory failure

    g) Metabolic disturbance (calcium, urea nitrogen, glucose, sodium)

    h) Nicotine, alcohol, drug withdrawal

    i) Extreme, uncontrolled anxiety

3.   Assess for

   a)   Confusion vs. delirium using available tools such as those listed below[5]

      i.   Memorial Delirium Assessment Scale (MDAS)

      ii.   Delirium Rating Scale (DRS)

      iii.   NEECHAM Confusion Scale (NCS)

      iv.   Confusion Assessment Method (CAM)

   b)   Differentiation between hyper-alert—hyperactive and hypo-alert—hypoactive variants of delirium

   c)   Patient's previous personality and emotional coping abilities

   d)   Alcohol, drug use history; recent nicotine, alcohol or drug use

   e)   Signs of infection

      i.   Fever, flushing, tachycardia, tachypnea, perspiration

      ii.   These symptoms of infection may not be present in persons with immunosuppression due to corticosteroids, chemotherapy, disease process or in the elderly

   f)   Abdominal examination: palpate for bladder or bowel, abdominal distention

   g)   Bowel history, noting time and character of last bowel movement; rectal examination for impaction

   h)   If diabetic history or currently on corticosteroids, capillary blood glucose

   i)   Lab studies including: BUN, creatinine, electrolytes, glucose, calcium

   j)   Consider midstream clean-catch urinalysis, culture and sensitivity

   k)   Neurologic status: dysphasia, weakness, bilateral strength, coordination; poor coordination

   l)   Patient safety

   m)   Patient and family coping with change in mental status and ways of managing patient

4.   Potential diagnoses

   a)   Altered mental status changes potentially related to (etiology)

   b)   High safety risk for fall related to altered mental status

   c)   Impaired bowel function related to constipation from (etiology)

   d)   Impaired bladder function related to retention from (etiology)

   e)   Disturbed physiologic response to infection related to corticosteroid use, aging

   f)   Impaired physiologic response related to alcohol, drugs, medication

   g)   Risk for alcohol, drug withdrawal due to recent use

5. Planning and Intervention

    a) Etiology of altered mental status will determine intervention plan

    b) Effective pain control and control of other disabling symptoms

    c) Assess patient's current medications for compliance, effects and iatrogenic effects (side effects) contributing to altered mental status

    d) Review with physician and/or pharmacist; consider discontinuation or reduction of medications thought to be contributing to patient's confusion

    e) Correct metabolic imbalance, if appropriate

    f) Support alcohol, drug withdrawal chemically as indicated

    g) Treat infection as appropriate

    h) For impaction, disimpact; establish aggressive bowel regimen

    i) For urine retention, straight or retention catheter to relieve

    j) Support withdrawal from nicotine, alcohol or drugs if withdrawal is contributing to agitation

    k) Reassure patient and family and provide constant, consistent reorientation of confused patient

    l) Provide for patient's safety; follow agency/institutional policy regarding the use of restraints, both chemical and physical

    m) Avoid sedation if possible

    n) Psychotropic drugs do not reverse confusion or altered mental status, but they may calm distressing agitation, paranoia or hallucinations

        i.   Haloperidol and chlorpromazine are first line medications

        ii. Risperidone is particularly helpful in managing agitation and hallucinations in the elderly

6. Patient and family education

    a) Since confusion is most distressing to patients and families, much education and support is required

    b) Intermittent nature of most confusion

    c) Expected therapeutic response to interventions

    d) Expected medication effects and potential side effects

    e) Safety needs of patient during periods of confusion, agitation

    f) Importance of compliance with bowel regimen, bladder emptying

7. Evaluate

    a) Effectiveness of interventions

        i.   Medications

        ii. Non-pharmacologic interventions

        b)   Family participation and coping

        c)   Reassess to determine additional needs

  8.   Revise plan according to findings from ongoing evaluations, changes in patient status or family needs

B. Terminal Restlessness

  1.   Definitions

        a)   Excessive restlessness, increased mental and physical activity[5]

        b)   Commonly seen features are frequent, non-purposeful motor activity, inability to concentrate or relax, disturbances in sleep or rest patterns, potential for progression to agitation[7]

  2.   Potential etiologies include

        a)   Full bladder, constipation/impaction

        b)   Hypoxia, dyspnea

        c)   Left ventricular failure, decreased cardiac output

        d)   Uncontrolled pain

        e)   Denial, anxiety, unfinished emotional, and/or spiritual issues

        f)   Also consider the possible etiologies listed above for confusion/delirium/agitation

  3.   Assess for

        a)   Etiology of terminal restlessness

        b)   Emotional, spiritual history related to issues, personal peace, resolution

        c)   Shortness of breath or labored breathing; lung sounds

        d)   Bladder and bowel status

        e)   Hallucinations, muscle twitching or jerking

        f)   "Sundowning"

  4.   Potential diagnoses

        a)   Disturbed mental status related to (etiology)

        b)   High risk for injury due to agitation and uncontrolled restlessness

        c)   Family coping impairment related to severe stress of uncontrolled agitation

  5.   Plan and interventions

        a)   Etiology of restlessness will determine intervention plan

        b)   Disimpaction, bladder relief if distended

    c)   Consult physician or pharmacist for pharmacologic management. Medications may include

        i.   Opioid analgesics for pain and sedation

        ii.   Antipsychotics

            (a)   ChlorproMAZINE

            (b)   Haloperidol

            (c)   Risperidone is particularly helpful in managing agitation and hallucinations in the elderly

        iii.   Barbiturates

            (a)   Phenobarbital

        iv.   Benzodiazepines

            (a)   Lorazepam (if no delirium, caution with dementia)

            (b)   Diazepam (caution with dementia)

            (c)   Midazolam

    d)   Medications should be given by the least invasive route possible: oral, rectal, transdermal, subcutaneous or intravenous; intramuscular route should be used only if absolutely necessary

    e)   Regular assessment of medication effects

    f)   Pharmacologic control of muscle twitching, jerking

    g)   Pastoral and psychological support of patient and family for emotional and spiritual issues

    h)   Non-pharmacologic approaches including

        i.   Subdued, quiet, calm environment

        ii.   Consistent, familiar faces and staff

        iii.   Calm and reassuring presence

        iv.   Relaxation techniques

            (a)   Visualization

            (b)   Distraction

            (c)   Massage

        v.   Pet therapy, if appropriate

        vi.   Aromatherapy

6. Family education

   a) Calm environment, presence with minimal stimulation

   b) Non-pharmacologic methods for cueing patient with relaxation, visualization, massage, music, distraction

   c) Expected therapeutic response to medications and potential side effects

   d) Prepare family for patient's sedation response to medications

   e) Prepare family for patient's death; encourage speaking with/to patient and using "letting go" language and phrases if family able

7. Evaluate

   a) Effectiveness of interventions

      i. Medications

      ii. Non-pharmacologic interventions

   b) Family participation and coping

   c) Reassess to determine additional needs

8. Revise plan according to findings from ongoing evaluations, changes in patient status or family needs

IV. Anorexia and Cachexia

A. Definitions

1. Anorexia: loss of appetite or inability to take in nutrients

2. Cachexia: weight loss and wasting due to inadequate intake of nutrients

B. Possible Etiologies

1. Anorexia

   a) Pain

   b) Constipation

   c) Nausea and vomiting

   d) Alteration in oral mucous membranes (candidiasis, xerostomia, mucositis)

   e) Impaired gastric emptying

   f) Change of taste in foods (dysgeusia); change in smell of foods

   g) Altered mental status (depression, dementia, confusion, anxiety)

   h) Fatigue

   i) Medications (opioids, antibiotics)

   j) Radiation or chemotherapy

2. Cachexia

    a) Increased nutritional losses related to etiologies associated with anorexia

    b) Increased nutritional losses associated with[3]

        i. Bleeding

        ii. Diarrhea

        iii. Malabsorption of nutrients (i.e., pancreatic cancer)

    c) Metabolic Disorders

        i. Abnormal protein metabolism (negative nitrogen balance and decreased muscle mass)

        ii. Abnormal carbohydrate metabolism due to inefficient energy metabolism

        iii. Abnormal lipid metabolism (overall depletion of total body fat)

        iv. Change in fluid and electrolyte balance (increase in extracellular fluid and total body sodium and decrease in intracellular fluid and total body potassium)[3]

C. Assess For

1. History of loss of appetite, including reasons for loss (i.e., change in taste or smell, dysphagia, nausea and vomiting)

2. Patient food likes and dislikes

3. Oral mucosa for dryness, sores, candidiasis

4. Medications that may cause a decrease in appetite

5. Symptoms of malabsorption, such as diarrhea

6. Decrease in bowel sounds

7. Signs and symptoms of constipation or fecal impaction

8. Signs and symptoms of metabolic disorder, such as hypoglycemia, hypernatremia, hypokalemia, dehydration, hypercalcemia

9. Patient/family knowledge of etiology of anorexia and cachexia

D. Potential Diagnoses

1. Nutrition less than body requirements related to anorexia

2. Fatigue, related to decreased nutritional intake secondary to anorexia

3. Body image disturbance, related to cachexia

4. Anxiety related to inability to eat as desired

5. Patient/family knowledge deficit related to etiology and management of anorexia/cachexia

E. **Plan/Interventions**[3]

   1. Encourage patient and family to prepare foods the patient likes and have those foods available whenever the patient requests them

   2. Refer to Interdisciplinary Team dietitian

   3. Give patient permission to eat less than before

   4. Encourage small, frequent meals rather than three large meals

   5. Avoid strong odors; allow food to cool before serving

   6. Serve small portions with a pleasing appearance

   7. In cases where anorexia is due to nausea/vomiting, altered oral mucous membranes, constipation or diarrhea (see sections II, X, XI in this chapter)

   8. Encourage nutritional supplements

   9. Enteral feedings may be appropriate in certain cases if patient's GI function is adequate for digestion/absorption

  10. Parenteral nutrition support (total or peripheral parenteral nutrition, i.e., TPN or PPN) if indicated and desired by patient/family (rare in hospice setting)

  11. Pharmacologic interventions (see Table 2)

F. **Patient/Family Education**

   1. Encourage patient to eat as often as desired, but assure patient it is okay not to eat if it is uncomfortable

   2. Explain dying process to patient/family, especially that anorexia is normal in last days of life

   3. Encourage open communication regarding nutrition

G. **Evaluate**

   1. Has patient's appetite and nutritional intake increased, if this was a goal?

   2. Patient/family response to interventions. Are they satisfied with outcome?

   3. Are symptoms contributing to anorexia/cachexia treated, if appropriate?

H. **Revise plan according to findings from ongoing evaluations, changes in patient status or family needs**

Table 2: Anorexia/Cachexia: Pharmacologic Interventions

Class of Drug	Example(s)	Comments
Gastrokinetic Agents	Metoclopramide 10 mg po tid	Useful in patients complaining of nausea or early satiety.
Corticosteroids	Dexamethasone 4 mg po q am, then taper gradually to the minimum effective dosage	Highly effective in improving appetite in the short term, with side effects at the dosage recommended; may lose efficacy after a few weeks.
Progesterone Analogs	Megestrol acetate 400–800 mg po qd Medroxy-PROGESTERone acetate 100 mg po tid	80% of patients will show improvement in appetite; significant decreases in nausea and vomiting occur in more than 50%; abnormalities of taste are often reduced, and weight gain (of fat, fluid and lean body mass) is seen in nearly all patients except those in the most terminal stages. Treatment with recommended dosage costs $2/day (more expensive but has fewer side effects than steroids).
Cannabinoids	Dronabinol 2.5 mg po bid 1 hour pc	An effective appetite stimulant in low doses, without the usual side effects of drowsiness and muddled thinking.
Alcohol	1 glass of beer or sherry before meals	May improve appetite and morale in patients who enjoyed a drink before dinner when they were well.
Vitamins	Multivitamins Vitamin C, 500 mg qid	Anecdotal evidence of improved appetite (may be due to placebo effect).

Reprinted from *Handbook of Palliative Care in Cancer*, 2nd ed., A. Waller and N. L. Caroline, p. 152, Copyright 2000 with permission from Elsevier.

V. Ascites

A. Definition: the accumulation of excessive fluid in the peritoneal cavity

B. Possible Etiologies

1. Portal hypertension: obstruction of portal vessels, causing leakage into abdominal cavity. Usually due to

    a) Cirrhosis

    b) Cancer (ovarian, endometrial, breast, colon, pancreatic, gastric, lymphoma, liver)

    c) Cardiac dysfunction: congestive heart failure, constrictive pericarditis

2. Decreased plasma oncotic pressure: decrease in plasma albumin levels, causing fluid to leave plasma and accumulate in abdomen. Usually due to

    a) Cirrhosis

    b) Nephrotic syndrome

    c) Malnutrition

3. Lymphatic obstruction due to tumor infiltration in the abdomen, causing a buildup of fluid in the abdomen

C. Assess For

1. History relating to etiology (i.e., liver damage, cancer, alcoholism)

2. Weight gain

3. Tachycardia, dyspnea, orthopnea

4. Decrease in mobility: unable to bend or sit straight

5. Peripheral edema

6. Abdominal signs

    a) Measure abdominal girth every visit

    b) Fluid wave test

    c) Shifting dullness test

    d) Abdominal striae

    e) Distended abdominal wall veins

7. Dehydration

8. Anorexia/early satiety

D.   **Diagnoses**

1.   Pain, related to increasing abdominal girth

2.   Immobility, and fatigue secondary to ascites

3.   Impaired gas exchange related to ascites

4.   Activity intolerance related to ascites

5.   Patient/family knowledge deficit related to etiology and treatment of ascites

E.   **Planning and Intervention**

1.   Treatment is determined by the extent of fluid accumulation

2.   Analgesics (usually low-dose opioids) can be used for the pain and discomfort of abdominal distention

3.   Fluid and sodium restriction: limit fluid to 500–1000 cc/day, and sodium to 200–1000 mg/day; may not be successful in malignant ascites[6]

4.   Diuretics may be added if fluid and sodium restriction has not been successful after four to five days; spironolactone (Aldactone®) is drug of choice, with furosemide (Lasix®) added with start of spironolactone or if spironolactone alone is not successful

5.   Paracentesis may be indicated for palliation if the patient's comfort is extremely compromised

6.   Palliative chemotherapy may reduce tumor size and invasion, which may be causing ascites

7.   Close monitoring of intake and output may be needed, depending on where patient is on disease trajectory

F.   **Patient/Family Education**

1.   Discuss dietary measures (fluid and sodium restriction) to reduce ascites

2.   Explain effects of medication and potential side effects (including dehydration for diuretics)

3.   Explain skin problems associated with ascites, and demonstrate proper measures for maintaining skin integrity

4.   Discuss signs and symptoms of infection if paracentesis is part of the treatment plan

G.   **Evaluate**

1.   Effectiveness of interventions and patient/family teaching (are patient/family satisfied with outcome?)

2.   Medication effectiveness and presence of side effects

3.   Skin integrity

H.   **Revise plan according to findings from ongoing evaluations, changes in patient status or family needs**

VI. Aphasia

A. Definition: absence or impairment of ability to communicate through speech, writing or signs

B. Possible Etiologies

1. Left cerebral hemisphere lesion from infarct, hemorrhage, tumor, trauma or degeneration

2. Advanced dementia, cerebral vascular disease

C. Assess For

1. Type of aphasia

    a) Sensory (receptive) aphasia: inability to comprehend spoken or written words

    b) Motor (expressive) aphasia: comprehension but inability or impairment of speech

    c) Global (sensory & motor) aphasia: failure of all forms of communication

2. Impairment of patient's ability to communicate pain, comfort needs

3. Difficulty in assessment of patient orientation, knowledge, judgment, abstraction, calculation ability and emotional responses, which can impact patient education, safety management

4. Caregiver's abilities, willingness to interpret patient's needs

5. Patient and family frustration, anxiety about deficits in communication

D. Potential Diagnoses

1. Speech and communication impairment related to type of aphasia and probable etiology

2. Compromised patient/family coping, stress, tolerance related to onset of aphasia

3. Patient knowledge deficit related to adjustment to impairment, disease process, therapeutic regimen related to aphasia

E. Planning and Intervention

1. Model acceptance and patience in communication

2. Speech therapy clinician consultation for recommendations for improving communication

3. Writing or picture boards for expressive aphasia

4. Ongoing inquiry and monitoring of patient's non-verbal behaviors for anxiety, pain, discomfort

5. Consistency in communication with patient from family and interdisciplinary team members

F.   **Patient/Family Education**

   1.   Instruct, support caregiver/family in learning patient's non-verbal cues and developing signs, signals for communicating patient's needs: e.g. pain relief, toileting, thirst, hunger, repositioning, emotional feelings

   2.   Instruct in reducing excessive stimuli in environment that can distract communication

G.   **Evaluate for effectiveness of interventions, specifically**

   1.   Development of alternate communication tools

   2.   Patient/family coping and adaptation

   3.   Patient comfort: symptom progression or relief (pain or other)

   4.   Patient needs being met

   5.   Interdisciplinary team consistency

H.   **Revise plan according to findings from ongoing evaluations, changes in patient status or family needs**

VII. Bladder Spasms

A.   **Definition: intermittent, painful contractions of the detrusor muscle, leading to suprapubic pain and urgency**

B.   **Possible Etiologies**

   1.   Indwelling catheter and/or problems associated with indwelling catheters (obstruction, size or balloon too large)

   2.   Urinary tract infection

   3.   Encroachment on bladder or urethra by tumor or impacted feces

   4.   Radiation or chemotherapy cystitis

   5.   Urethral obstruction by tumors or blood clots

   6.   Neurologic disorders: stroke, spinal cord lesions, multiple sclerosis

C.   **Assess For**

   1.   Possible etiologies as documented in the medical history (history of bladder or prostate cancer, neurologic disorders, recent radiation or chemotherapy)

   2.   Signs and symptoms of urinary tract infection

   3.   Indwelling catheter function, assess catheter and balloon size as possible source of spasm

   4.   Hematuria

   5.   Food and fluid intake: some foods aggravate symptoms; adequate fluid intake important for urinary tract health

   6.   Presence of fecal impaction

D. Potential Diagnoses

1. Pain related to bladder spasm secondary to obstruction/infection/disease process

2. Altered urinary elimination related to bladder spasm

3. Patient and family knowledge deficit related to disease process, management of indwelling catheter, and treatment of bladder spasm

E. Planning and Intervention: Etiology will guide treatment

1. Presence of indwelling catheter

    a) Reassess the need for Foley catheter

    b) Change catheter to appropriate size

    c) Partially deflate balloon

    d) Gently irrigate with normal saline

    e) May need to initiate continuous saline irrigation if etiology is related to blood clots

2. Urinary tract infection

    a) Antibiotics

    b) Reassess the need for Foley catheter

    c) Change catheter if catheterized

    d) Increase oral fluid intake if feasible

3. Disimpact if etiology is fecal impaction

4. Non-pharmacologic measures: assisting the patient to void every 4 hours, sitting or standing to void, teach relaxation techniques

5. Pharmacologic measures: antispasmodic drugs such as oxybutynin (Ditropan®); NSAIDs; Belladonna and Opium (B & O) suppositories, hyoscyamine

F. Patient/Family Education

1. Explain etiology of bladder spasm and measures to reduce symptoms

2. Demonstrate proper catheter care and explain signs and symptoms of catheter obstruction

3. Explain signs and symptoms of urinary tract infection

4. Teach expected medication effects and potential side effects

G. Evaluate

1. Effectiveness of interventions and/or medications in decreasing pain related to bladder spasm

2. Effectiveness of antibiotic therapy, if appropriate

3. Patient/family understanding of interventions and medication regimen and recognition of symptoms

  H. **Revise plan according to findings from ongoing evaluations, changes in patient status or family needs**

VIII. Bowel Incontinence

  A. **Definition: the inability to control bowel movements**

  B. **Possible Etiologies**

    1. Obstruction, including fecal impaction or tumor (overflow incontinence)

    2. Diarrhea (see Section XI: Diarrhea)

    3. Sphincter damage due to rectal carcinoma, recto-vaginal fistula, or inflammatory bowel disease involving the rectum

    4. Sensory or motor dysfunction of the rectosphincter due to spinal cord lesions or compression, multiple sclerosis, diabetes

    5. Changes in sphincter tone related to age or spinal cord compression

    6. Dementia or mobility related (unable to verbalize or recognize need or unable to reach the toilet)

  C. **Assess For**

    1. Rectal urgency and passage of loose or formed stool without patient control; incontinence of formed stool usually related to dementia[7], fecal impaction

    2. Functional status: is patient able to reach toilet?

    3. Neurologic and sensory function

    4. Skin integrity

  D. **Potential Diagnoses**

    1. Bowel incontinence related to obstruction, diarrhea, neurosensory dysfunction, or impaired cognition

    2. Risk for impaired skin integrity related to bowel incontinence

    3. Patient/family knowledge deficit related to etiology and management of bowel incontinence

    4. Patient/family anxiety related to bowel incontinence

  E. **Planning and Intervention: Etiology will guide interventions**

    1. Review bowel regimen and adjust laxative dose as needed if patient is taking opioids for pain

    2. Utilize opioids for constipating effect (codeine most effective)

    3. Disimpact if fecal impaction is causing incontinence; may need opioid or anxiolytic prior to disimpaction

4. Modify dietary practices if appropriate and as tolerated

 a) Decrease fiber intake to reduce bulk formation of stool

 b) Increase fluid intake of lukewarm, room temperature, or cool beverages (very cold or hot liquids can act as stimulants)

 c) Avoid spicy, greasy, rich, and fried foods; avoid caffeine and high amounts of milk products

 d) Incorporate bananas, rice, applesauce into diet; eat several small frequent meals rather than large meals

5. Alter environment to place patient closer to toileting facilities

6. Initiate a bowel routine (i.e., taking patient to toilet after eating)

7. Maintain skin integrity with adequate skin cleansing and liberal use of skin protectant ointment

8. Utilize incontinence products

F. Patient/Family Education

1. Explain etiology of bowel incontinence, and appropriate interventions relative to the etiology

2. Explain effects of medication and potential side effects

3. Demonstrate correct hygiene and skin care techniques to prevent skin breakdown

4. Explain safety measures if altering environment for ease in toileting (i.e., have patient call for assistance, bowel routine, assuring clear path to bathroom)

G. Evaluate

1. Effectiveness of interventions and patient/family teaching (Are patient/family satisfied with outcome?)

2. Medication effectiveness and presence of side effects.

3. Skin integrity

4. Patient safety

H. Revise plan according to findings from ongoing evaluations, changes in patient status or family needs

IX. Bowel Obstruction

A. Definition: occlusion of the lumen of the intestine, delaying or preventing the normal passage of feces

B.   **Possible Etiologies**

1.   External compression of the lumen (i.e., tumor enlargement, metastases, adhesions, organomegaly)

2.   Internal occlusion of the lumen (i.e., tumor, intussusception)

3.   Ischemic or inflammatory processes (i.e., Crohn's disease, diverticulitis, peritonitis, pancreatitis, hernia)

4.   Fecal blockage (severe constipation can mimic obstruction)

5.   Adynamic ileus (i.e., pneumonia, metabolic/electrolyte problems)

6.   Metabolic disorders (i.e., Crohn's disease, hypokalemia)

7.   Drugs (i.e., diuretics can cause hypokalemia, which decreases peristalsis; opioids; chemotherapy)

8.   Often more than one etiology is present when a bowel obstruction develops

C.   **Assess For**

1.   History: predisposition to obstruction (cancer, pancreatitis, etc.), history of bowel habits, medication usage, history of pain

2.   Pain

   a)   Crampy, colicky pain in the middle to upper abdomen relieved with vomiting suggests a small bowel obstruction

   b)   Crampy pain in the lower abdomen that increases over time suggests a large bowel obstruction

   c)   Severe, steady pain is a sign of bowel strangulation

3.   Abdominal Distention: present and possibly severe in obstruction of the large intestine; visible peristalsis may be present; patient may complain of constipation and bloating

4.   Nausea and Vomiting: moderate to severe in small bowel obstruction and can relieve pain. May develop later in obstruction of the large intestine

5.   Bowel sounds: hyperactive sounds and borborygmi; hypoactive or absent sounds with adynamic ileus

6.   Constipation and inability to pass flatus seen in complete obstruction

7.   Diarrhea due to overflow of feces related to fecal impaction

8.   Fever and chills could indicate bowel ischemia or strangulation

D.   **Possible Diagnoses**

1.   Pain related to bowel obstruction

2.   Potential for fluid and electrolyte imbalances related to vomiting secondary to bowel obstruction

3.   Anxiety related to pain and inability to defecate secondary to bowel obstruction

4.   Nausea and vomiting related to bowel obstruction

5.   Patient/family knowledge deficit related to etiology and treatment of bowel obstruction

E. Planning and Intervention

1. Disimpact if necessary, utilizing an opioid or anxiolytic if needed for patient comfort

2. Surgery may be considered if

    a) This is patient's first obstruction

    b) The obstruction occurs in only one site

    c) The patient's prognosis and condition will allow for a good outcome[8]

    d) Surgery is not usually indicated for non-mechanical obstructions

3. Medication for pain including antispasmodics (loperamide or scopolamine), and opioids

4. Stimulant laxatives (senna, bisacodyl) and prokinetics (metoclopramide) should be discontinued if patient is experiencing colicky pain or complete bowel obstruction[8]

5. Medication for nausea and vomiting (if symptoms are distressful for patient) including promethazine, prochlorperazine, or haloperidol

6. Gastric decompression using NG suction may be necessary for relief of gastric distention and nausea; if symptoms persist, percutaneous gastrostomy placement can aid in venting

7. Oral fluids should be increased if tolerable and nausea and vomiting can be controlled; parenteral fluids may be considered if vomiting is not controlled and patient at risk for severe dehydration

8. Treat diarrhea or constipation according to interventions outlined in sections X and XI

F. Patient/Family Education

1. Explain etiology and treatment course of bowel obstruction

2. Explain medication effects and possible side effects

3. Demonstrate post-operative care of incisions/gastrostomy tube, if appropriate

4. Explain importance of bowel regimen, and assist in initiating regimen, if appropriate

G. Evaluate

1. Effectiveness of interventions and patient/family teaching

2. Effects and side effects of medications

3. Patient/family understanding of treatment and prevention of further obstruction

H. Revise plan according to findings from ongoing evaluations, changes in patient status or family needs

X. Constipation

A. **Definition: difficulty in passing stools or an incomplete or infrequent passage of hard stools**

B. **Possible Etiologies**

1. Intestinal obstruction: tumors in bowel wall, external compression of the bowel by pelvic or abdominal tumors

2. Medications: opioids, tricyclic antidepressants, phenothiazines, antacids, diuretics, iron, vincristine, anti-hypertensives, anticonvulsants, anticholinergics or drugs with anticholinergic effects, NSAIDs

3. Metabolic disorders: hypercalcemia, hypokalemia, hypothyroidism

4. Other disease processes or disorders: colitis, diverticular disease

5. Dietary problems: low fiber intake, inadequate fluid intake, dehydration

6. Neurologic: confusion, depression, sedation

7. Weakness, inactivity, and immobility

8. Pain associated with constipation, including anal fissures or hemorrhoids, straining at stool, etc.

9. Decrease in privacy or unfamiliar toilet facilities; patient reluctant to ask for help in toileting (embarrassment, loss of independence, do not want to be a burden, etc.)

C. **Assess For**

1. Bowel history

    a) Last bowel movement and bowel movement prior to last

    b) Amount, color, consistency

    c) Straining or pain during defecation

    d) Current bowel regimen: does patient need aids in defecation, such as laxatives, suppositories, or digital removal

2. Food and fluid intake

3. Mobility potential

4. Abdominal assessment: abdominal distension and/or tenderness; may report feeling of fullness or bloating; bowel sounds may be normal or hypoactive; percussion reveals dullness in otherwise tympanic areas; may be able to palpate stool in colon

5. Increase in flatus

6. Nausea, vomiting

7. Rectal examination: presence of hemorrhoids, anal fissures; digital examination might reveal hard stool or large amount of soft stool in rectum

8. Patient/family understanding of underlying cause of constipation, expected effects of medication or non-pharmacological remedies

D. **Potential Diagnoses**

1. Risk for constipation related to opioid or other constipating medication usage, immobility, decrease in food, fluid intake

2. Constipation related to opioid medication usage, immobility, decrease in food, fluid intake

3. Alteration in comfort related to constipation

4. Patient/family knowledge deficit related to appropriate bowel regimen

E. **Planning and Intervention**

1. Goal in control of opioid-induced constipation is prevention of constipation

2. Bowel obstruction should be ruled out and disimpaction considered if appropriate

    a) If digitally disimpacting, give an opioid or anxiolytic prior to intervention

    b) Digital disimpaction contraindicated in neutropenic or thrombocytopenic patients; may be contraindicated in end stage cardiac patients

3. Non-pharmacologic therapies

    a) Increase fluid intake: water and fruit juices are most effective (prune juice is especially helpful)

    b) Encourage high-fiber foods; examples include: whole grain breads and cereals, bran cereal, fresh, canned, frozen or dried fruits and vegetables

    c) Increase activity, including active or passive range of motion if possible

    d) Ask patient what has been effective in the past

4. Pharmacologic therapies

    a) If patient is at risk for constipation, prophylactic stool softener and stimulant laxatives should be started (example: Peri-Colace® or senna with docusate sodium)[9]

    b) Patient may use own regimen, but regular use should be stressed, especially if using opioids

    c) If no bowel movement in three days, regardless of intake, fluids should be increased and an osmotic laxative (i.e., lactulose, sorbitol) started

    d) For continuing constipation, a glycerin or bisacodyl suppository or sodium biphosphate enema may be added[9]

    e) Discontinue medications that may cause constipation if not medically necessary (i.e., iron or calcium supplements)

5. Rectal pain or discomfort: consider hemorrhoid preparations or warm sitz baths (rule out herpes in the case of a patient with HIV disease)

F. **Patient/Family Education**

1. Explain etiology of constipation and instruct in ways to manage

    a) Non-pharmacological interventions: increased food/fluid intake, increase activity

    b) Pharmacological interventions

2.   Continually reinforce necessity of bowel regime, even if patient is not constipated

3.   Explain medication effects and possible side effects

4.   Reinforce that bowel movement should occur at least every three days, and further action should be taken if no bowel movement after this time

G.   Evaluate

1.   Effectiveness of bowel regime

    a)   How often is patient having bowel movement?

    b)   Is patient having difficulty during passage of stool?

2.   Assess abdomen and rectum (externally and digitally, if appropriate)

3.   Patient/family understanding of bowel regime, including medications and non-pharmacologic measures to prevent constipation

H.   Revise plan according to findings from ongoing evaluations, changes in patient status, or family needs

XI.   Diarrhea

A.   Definition: the frequent passage of loose, unformed, liquid stool

B.   Possible Etiologies

1.   Laxative therapy overuse or imbalance

2.   Side effect of other drugs (i.e., NSAIDs, antibiotics)

3.   Radiation and chemotherapy

4.   Food intolerances or tube feedings

5.   Malnutrition (cachexia related to cancer or AIDS)

6.   Surgical procedures: gastrectomy, ileal resection, colectomy

7.   Fecal impaction

8.   Infection (especially as seen in immunocompromised patients, such as those with AIDS and post-chemotherapy)

9.   Partial intestinal obstruction

10.   Tumors: gastrointestinal and carcinoid tumors, pancreatic islet cell tumors, small cell lung tumors

11.   Gastrointestinal disorders: inflammatory bowel disease, pancreatic insufficiency, diverticulitis, ulcerative colitis, Crohn's disease

12.   Other chronic disorders such as diabetes and hyperthyroidism

C. **Assessment**

1. History, including characteristic of stool, how often stool is occurring, medication usage, recent radiation or chemotherapy treatments or gastrointestinal surgery

2. Physical exam

a) Abdominal assessment: bowel sounds may be hyperactive (or hypoactive to absent if intestinal obstruction is present), patient reports of cramping or pain, palpable masses in abdomen may indicate partial obstruction

b) Nature and consistency of stool (if available to assess): pancreatic insufficiency is indicated by steatorrhea (loose, pale, foul-smelling, greasy stool); fecal impaction may be indicated by small amounts of loose stool

3. Signs of dehydration

4. Skin integrity

D. **Potential Diagnoses**

1. Diarrhea related to infection, metabolic disorders, medications or therapies, partial obstruction, malnutrition, or GI intolerance to food/feedings

2. Risk for impaired skin integrity related to diarrhea

3. Potential for fluid and electrolyte imbalance related to diarrhea

4. Patient/family knowledge deficit related to etiology and treatment of diarrhea

E. **Planning and Intervention: Etiology will guide treatment options**

1. Increase fluid intake, preferably with electrolyte replacement drinks

2. Clear liquid diet for first 24 hours, with light carbohydrates (rice, crackers, etc.), then advance as tolerated to diet high in protein and calories; avoid spicy, greasy, high-fiber foods and foods high in lactose or caffeine; small, frequent meals are usually better tolerated. Incorporate bananas, rice, applesauce into diet to help keep stool firm in consistency

3. Disimpact if necessary, utilizing opioids or anxiolytics prior to intervention, if needed for patient comfort

4. Discontinue laxatives if certain etiology of diarrhea is not due to impaction

5. Antidiarrheals: loperamide; diphenoxylate HCl with atropine (absorbent and adsorbent agents do not work as fast, so are not indicated in advanced disease); opioids can also be considered if patient is not already taking

6. Pancreatic insufficiency: pancreatic enzymes with meals, with loperamide (slows peristalsis)

7. Maintain skin integrity with adequate skin cleansing and liberal use of skin protectant ointment

F.   Patient/Family Education

1.   Explain etiology of diarrhea, and appropriate interventions relative to the etiology

2.   Explain effects of medication and potential side effects

3.   Demonstrate correct hygiene and skin care techniques to prevent skin breakdown

4.   Explain signs, symptoms and treatment of dehydration

G.   Evaluate

1.   Effectiveness of interventions and patient/family teaching (are patient/family satisfied with outcome?)

2.   Medication effectiveness and presence of side effects

3.   Skin integrity

4.   Fluid volume status

H.   Revise plan according to findings from ongoing evaluations, changes in patient status or family needs

XII. Dysphagia/Odynophagia

A.   Dysphagia: a subjective awareness of difficulty in swallowing

1.   Possible etiologies[2]

   a)   Obstructive: cancer of esophagus and other cancers of the head and neck area, benign peptic stricture & lower esophageal ring (history of GERD [Gastroesophageal Reflux Disease]), compression of vessels or mediastinal nodes. This type of dysphagia is intermittent, usually occurring when eating or drinking; solid foods are most difficult foods to swallow; some patients can tolerate only liquids

   b)   Motor: neuromuscular, esophageal dysfunction (stasis) related to smooth muscle hypertonia or dystonia: e.g., cardiospasm, esophageal aperistalsis, diffuse esophageal spasm (GERD), amyotrophic lateral sclerosis, Parkinson's disease, multiple sclerosis and dementia; this type of dysphagia is often for both solids and liquids

   c)   Systemic dysphagia: scleroderma, inflammation and infections affect swallowing ability

   d)   General deconditioning: chronic diseases can cause fatigue and general deconditioning

      i.   Medications that can contribute to dysphagia include anticholinergics, tricyclic antidepressants, antipsycotics and neuroleptic medications by causing dryness, slowing esophageal peristalsis and decreasing swallowing coordination

B.   Odynophagia: is a report of painful swallowing

    1.   Odynophagia possible etiologies

        a)   Inflammatory process: candidiasis, conditions favoring overgrowth of fungal *Candida albicans* e.g., broad spectrum antibiotics, diabetes mellitus, compromised cellular immunity (AIDS, leukemia, chemotherapy)

        b)   Dry mucous membranes due to xerostomia (decreased quantity or quality of saliva) from radiotherapy, anticholinergic or other medications

        c)   Corrosive esophagitis (ingestion of substance damaging to mucosa)

        d)   Bronchoesophageal fistula with chief complaint: "coughing after ingesting fluids"

C.   Assess For

    1.   Etiology of dysphagia or odynophagia, which will direct intervention plan

    2.   If odynophagia only, treatment of underlying cause may relieve symptom

        a)   Assess oral cavity including tongue, gingiva, mucosa, lips, presence and amount of saliva

        b)   Note onset and duration of painful swallowing

        c)   Assess voice quality, swallowing ability, oral hygiene

        d)   Oral intake: review 24 hour quantity food/liquid

        e)   Review history for AIDS, diabetes, chemotherapy, radiotherapy

        f)   Review current medications for contributing agents (steroid inhalers, steroids, antibiotics, sulfa)

        g)   Presence of creamy white curd-like patches in oropharynx, tongue; patches usually scrape off easily with 4x4 gauze; may cause bleeding

    3.   Current nutritional status related to disease process, goals of therapies, patient and family expectations

    4.   If dysphagia, odynophagia are accompanied by anorexia, evaluate patient for disease progression, current nutritional status; discuss management options with interdisciplinary team, patient and family

D.   Potential Diagnoses

    1.   Swallowing impairment, nutritional impairment related to dysphagia (amount of time) or odynophagia (amount of time)

    2.   Oral mucous membranes impairment related to: candidiasis, mucositis, xerostomia

    3.   Patient/family knowledge deficit of: nutrition; types of food, liquids; safety in food selection, expected medication, therapy effects and side effects

E. **Planning and Intervention**

1. If candidiasis: antifungal swish and swallow QID X 7–10 days; OR antifungal po X 5–7days

2. If mucositis or esophagitis from radiotherapy: topical anesthetic, antihistamine, antacid combination e.g. lidocaine/ diphenhydrAMINE/ antacid in 1:1:1 ratio as swish and swallow IF patient has gag reflex

3. If obstruction from tumors/nodes: limited dose steroids may reduce inflammatory edema

4. If neuro-motor etiology: speech therapy consult may be helpful to evaluate swallow and make recommendation

5. If dry mucosa induced from medications or radiotherapy: artificial saliva, lip balm, exquisite oral care, increase hydration

6. Determine food consistency best tolerated by patient: liquids may have thickening agents added to facilitate swallowing

7. If medications are etiology of dysphagia or odynophagia, consider alternative medicines if appropriate

8. Artificial feeding may be considered for obstructive or fistula processes in some palliative care situations depending upon the patient's place on the disease trajectory, current nutritional and functional status and other factors

F. **Patient/Family Education**

1. Importance of excellent oral hygiene

2. Avoid nicotine, alcohol and caffeine, which increase esophageal and vasospasm and have mucosal drying effects

3. Cool, non-irritating foods and liquids generally better tolerated

4. Encourage patient to chew food well and to avoid large boluses of meat, bread; modify food consistency if necessary, e.g., ground or pureed meats

5. Anticipated medication effects and potential side effects

G. **Evaluate for effectiveness of interventions, specifically**

1. Resolution of candidiasis

2. Improvement in mucosal lubrication

3. Oral hygiene

4. Nutritional status

5. Patient/family understanding of instructions, recommendations

H. **Revise plan according to findings from ongoing evaluations, changes in patient status or family needs**

XIII. Dyspnea/Cough

A. Definitions

1. Dyspnea: subjective sensation of shortness of breath

2. Cough: a natural defense of the body to prevent entry of foreign material into the respiratory tract[10]

B. Possible Etiologies

1. Dyspnea: lung tumor or metastases, pleural effusion, COPD, CHF, ascites, pneumothorax, pulmonary embolism, anemia, neurologic insult

2. Cough: infection, inflammation, cardiac (left ventricular failure), pulmonary disease (pleural effusion, bronchospasm, bronchogenic cancer), medications (ACE inhibitors), smoke, tobacco abuse or irritation from second-hand smoke, allergic conditions, GERD

C. Assess For

1. Dyspnea: etiology will direct intervention plan

    a) Onset of dyspnea, respiratory rate, depth, quality of respiration, lung sounds, accessory muscle use, stridor

    b) Past interventions that have provided relief/comfort

    c) Appropriate use and understanding of current medications for relief of dyspnea and accompanying anxiety

    d) Whether patient is a carbon dioxide (CO_2) retainer; this will influence decisions regarding oxygen delivery rate, opioid and anxiolytic dosing

    e) Patient/family anxiety, coping, understanding of dyspnea triggers and etiology, and interventions to control dyspnea

2. Cough: etiology will direct intervention plan

    a) History and physical to determine etiology and appropriate treatment

        i.   Productive vs. nonproductive cough

        ii. If productive, sputum quantity and appearance

        iii. Diagnostic studies as appropriate

    b) Effect of cough on patient/family's quality of life

    c) Need for cough suppressant OR cough expectorant based on etiology and patient need

D. Potential Diagnoses

1. Respiratory alteration related to: impairment of airway clearance, breathing pattern, or gas exchange

2. Patient/family knowledge deficit of: etiology or triggers of dyspnea and/or cough, steps to relieve dyspnea or anxiety; medication use, effects or side effects

3. Patient discomfort related to inability to control cough and/or mobilize secretions

4. Patient/family anxiety related to perceived situational powerlessness, fear, breathing impairment

E. Planning and Intervention[10]

1. Review of medical history, progression of disease, current medications; etiology of dyspnea will direct intervention plan

2. Non-pharmacologic interventions

    a) Dyspnea

        i. Position patient in high Fowler's position as appropriate; COPD patients do better leaning forward with upper arms supported on a table

        ii. Encourage pursed lip breathing in COPD patients

        iii. Palliative thoracentesis or paracentesis may be considered in selected patients

        iv. Model calm reassurance

        v. Encourage intake of nutrient-dense beverages (e.g., commercial supplements) if oral intake is limited because of dyspnea; liquids take less eating effort

        vi. Fan directly in front of patient; cool room environment

        vii. Complementary therapies such as relaxation techniques, guided imagery, therapeutic touch

        viii. Oxygen as appropriate

    b) Productive cough: chest physiotherapy (if able to tolerate), oxygen, humidity and suctioning, elevate head of bed, frequent sips of water, throat lozenges

3. Pharmacologic interventions

    a) Dyspnea and productive cough

        i. Opioids (PO, SL, SQ, IV or nebulized) for bronchodilatation

            (a) Start low (e.g., 5 mg po q2hr, prn) and titrate dose slowly for opioid-naïve patients and patients with CO_2 retention

            (b) Monitor respiratory rate and depth

        ii. High dose steroids for obstructive or inflammatory etiologies

        iii. Antibiotics for infection if appropriate

        iv. Anxiolytic medications may help to reduce the anxiety that often accompanies dyspnea: use and titrate slowly in elderly, dementia patients and patients with CO_2 retention; monitor respiratory rate and depth

        v. For uncontrolled dyspnea in hospice home-care setting, may consider short-term inpatient management

        vi. Sedation at end of life for refractory dyspnea is an option

b) Nonproductive cough: non-opioid (dextromethorphan, benzonatate) or opioid antitussives, inhaled anesthetic (lidocaine, bupivacaine)

    i. Nebulized lidocaine (e.g. 1%–5 ml) for 10 minutes q 2–6 hours

    ii. NPO for 1 hour post treatment due to risk of aspiration from loss of gag reflex from anesthetic agent

F. Patient/Family Education

1. Reassurance and empowerment of patient/family by review, rehearsal of steps to take when patient's shortness of breath begins

2. Treatment options, medication effects, side effects

3. Demonstrate relaxation techniques when patient/family is not in crisis

4. Instruct others not to crowd dyspneic person and to remain calm, in control of emotions

5. Consistency in information with rehearsal, review by all members of the interdisciplinary team

G. Evaluate

1. Understanding, compliance and effectiveness of medications for dyspneic episodes

2. For patient/family coping; reduction of, improvement in management and control of dyspneic episodes

3. For progression of disease process related to uncontrolled dyspnea

H. Revise plan according to findings from ongoing evaluations, changes in patient status or family needs

XIV. Edema

A. Definition: presence of excessive fluid in the intercellular tissues especially in the subcutaneous tissues

B. Possible Etiologies

1. Protein deficiency

2. Obstruction of venous return: peritoneal tumors, DVT, CHF, superior vena cava syndrome (SVC)

3. Renal failure

4. Lymphedema: blockage of lymphatic return in the periphery or the abdomen from surgical procedures, pressure from tumor

5. Ascites of liver failure; peritoneal inflammation

C.   Assess For

1.   Review of medical history and progression of disease process

2.   Etiology of edema, which will direct intervention plan

3.   New, increased or returning edema

4.   Extremity edema, pitting, non-pitting, tissue perfusion, warmth, cold, presence or absence of leaking from tissues

5.   Superior Vena Cava Syndrome (SVC)

   a)   Upper body edema, i.e., papilledema, facial edema, distended neck veins, one or both arms depending on where the obstruction is located: note onset, tissues involved

   b)   Other symptoms: dyspnea (most common), headache, chest pain, dry cough, visual or mental status changes, dizziness, vertigo

   c)   SVC is considered an oncologic emergency and may be palliated with radiotherapy with or without steroids depending on the etiology

   d)   Not responsive to diuretics

6.   Ascites: abdomen size, tenderness, distention, fluid wave; if elevated diaphragm, may have dyspnea, pleural effusion

7.   Patient/family understanding of disease process related to poor perfusion, expected medication effects and possible side effects

D.   Potential Diagnoses

1.   Tissue perfusion alteration related to: peripheral edema, ascites, upper body, head and neck edema

2.   Skin integrity impairment and risk related to poor perfusion, subcutaneous tissue edema, increased pressure points

3.   Respiratory alteration related to gas exchange impairment (for dyspnea related to ascites, SVC syndrome)

4.   Patient/family knowledge deficit of disease process, expected medication effects or possible side effects, non-pharmacologic measures

E.   Planning and Intervention

1.   Etiology of edema will direct intervention plan

2.   Symptomatic relief of ascites: spironolactone, paracentesis; the success of the diuretics in reducing ascites depends on the cause of the ascites[11]

3.   Symptomatic relief of peripheral edema: compression stockings; diuretics usually appropriate when there are also crackles heard in lungs; meticulous skin care; active or passive exercise to help venous return if patient can tolerate; limb elevation above level of heart

    4.   Lymphedema

        a)   Does not respond to diuretics unless there is a true peripheral edema component

        b)   May not resolve despite elevation, compression stockings

        c)   In the palliative care patient not actively dying, manual lymph drainage therapies may promote better quality of life

F.   Patient/Family Education

    1.   Explain etiology of edema and instruct in ways to manage or reduce

    2.   Expected medication effects and possible side effects

    3.   Application of compression stockings prior to ambulation

    4.   Post paracentesis care

G.   Evaluate

    1.   Effectiveness of medication

    2.   For level, return, extension of edema

    3.   Patient/family understanding of disease process, medications, application and use of compression stockings and/or manual lymph drainage therapies; non-pharmacologic interventions

H.   Revise plan according to findings from ongoing evaluations, changes in patient status or family needs

XV. Extrapyramidal Symptoms (EPS)

A.   Definition: involuntary movements, hyperkinetic (akathisia) or hypokinetic (dystonia); tardive dyskinesia is a late-effect, which may not respond to reversal therapies

B.   Possible Etiologies

    1.   Iatrogenic drug-induced from

        a)   Neuroleptics

        b)   Phenothiazines: e.g., chlorpromazine

        c)   Butyrophenones: e.g., haloperidol

        d)   Clozapine

        e)   Metoclopramide

        f)   Opioids (myoclonus)

    2.   Parkinson's disease, chorea

    3.   Cerebral lesions

C. **Assess For**

1. Etiology of EPS from medical history, medication review which will direct intervention plan

2. Possible iatrogenic response to a medical therapy used to treat a symptom

3. Patient safety with ambulation, activities of daily living (ADLs)

4. Patient/family anxiety relating to EPS, understanding of medication effects and side effects

D. **Diagnosis**

1. Impaired physical mobility related to neurologic impairment caused by: etiology

2. Self-care deficit related to: immobility, hyperactivity, loss of coordination

3. Patient/family knowledge deficit related to: medication effects or side effects, safety needs

E. **Planning and Intervention**

1. For phenothiazine toxicity

   a) Stop phenothiazine

   b) Benztropine mesylate (Cogentin®, trihexyphenidyl, or diphenhydrAMINE)

2. For akathisia (inability to sit still, pacing, agitation, restless movements)

   a) Benzodiazepines (lorazepam, diazepam)

   b) Beta-blockers (propranolol)

3. For dystonia, slow, retarded movements: physical or occupational therapy may be an adjunct if appropriate according to patient's place in the disease process, trajectory

4. In elderly, or others who may have sensitivity to anticholinergics: amantadine

5. Review of symptoms being treated with medication that may cause EPS; if symptoms remain present, discussion with medical team regarding alternative medications to control

F. **Patient/Family Education**

1. Stopping medication that may be contributing to EPS

2. Expected medication effects and potential side effects

3. Monitoring patient activity; safety in ambulation

G. **Evaluate for effectiveness of interventions, specifically**

1. Effect of medication change on EPS symptoms

2. Patient/family compliance, comfort with new medications

3. Control of symptoms

H. **Revise plan according to findings from ongoing evaluations, changes in patient status or family needs**

XVI. Hematologic Symptoms

A. Definitions

1. Hemorrhage: excessive bleeding

2. Clotting: systemic response to disease or medication that initiates coagulation cascade causing clotting

3. Cytopenia: reduction in bone marrow blood cell components, which can precipitate a systemic response

    a) Neutropenia: reduction in white blood cells; decreases patient's ability to respond to infection

    b) Thrombocytopenia: reduction in platelets; increases potential for frank, uncontrolled bleeding

    c) Anemias: reduction in production or maturation of red blood cells; low hemoglobin; decreased oxygen carrying cells; increased dyspnea, fatigue

    d) Pancytopenia: reduction in all blood cells

B. Possible Etiologies

1. Initiating coagulation cascade: deep vein thrombosis (DVT)

2. Immunologic processes (AIDS), drug-induced processes, prosthetic cardiac valves, veno-occlusive liver disease initiating coagulation cascade: hemorrhage, disseminated intravascular coagulopathy (DIC)

3. Chemotherapy, radiotherapy or disorders of spleen: thrombocytopenia, pancytopenia

4. Tumor erosion of blood vessels: hemorrhage

5. Pulmonary embolism (PE)

C. Assess For

1. Review medical history and current medications for potential hematology problems

2. Review current medications, foods, herbals for interactions with anticoagulant therapy

3. For DIC: petechiae, ecchymosis, oozing blood from mucous membranes, body orifices, puncture sites, signs of decreased perfusion to brain, kidneys, gastrointestinal, cardiovascular and peripheral vascular systems, lungs

4. For DVT: possible peripheral phlebitis, noting vascular access devices, streaking, erythema, heat over vein

5. For pulmonary embolism: sudden onset dyspnea

6. For thrombocytopenia: periorbital petechiae, epistaxis, gingival bleeding, blood-streaked sputum, emesis, urine or stool; acute shortness of breath, inspiratory pain, vaginal bleeding, petechiae, ecchymosis, joint pain, change in mental status, paresthesias

7. Patient/family understanding of and coping with changes in blood clotting response or pancytopenia; non-pharmacologic therapies, safety

D. Potential Diagnoses

1. Injury risk due to altered clotting patterns related to etiology

2. Infection risk due to neutropenia and body's reduced ability to control or fight infection

3. Patient/family knowledge deficit related to expected medication effects or side effects, safety needs, e.g. injury or infection

4. Medication risk related to anticoagulant therapy and other medications, herbals, foods

E. Plan and Intervention: treat underlying problem if appropriate

1. For DVT: anticoagulant therapy; monitor for other medications, foods and herbals that may interfere with anticoagulant therapy; anti-embolic stockings

2. For PE: anticoagulant therapy; monitor other medications, food and herbals that may interfere with anticoagulant therapy; anti-embolic stockings, treatment of dyspnea, pain

3. For Thrombocytopenia

   a) If palliative care: bleeding precautions, platelet transfusion for platelets <10,000, if appropriate

   b) If hospice: bleeding precautions, treat bleeding with compression, other non-pharmacologic interventions

4. For DIC: replenish clotting factors, e.g. platelets, fresh frozen plasma, antithrombin factor in palliative care; patient should be in an acute care facility for ongoing monitoring during therapy

5. For neutropenia: institute precautions against introduction of bacteria, infections to patient

6. Patient/family support, instruction, reassurance during bleeding and in anticipation of bleed

F. Patient/Family Education

1. Bleeding precautions

   a) Soft toothbrush and gentle motions for tooth brushing

   b) Care when using eating utensils

   c) Rinses for mouth

   d) No suppositories

   e) Safety in ambulation; prevent falls, injury

   f) Use electric razor rather than straight razor

2. For active bleed: long pressure for active bleed; use of dark towels; whom to call

3. For PE: elevate head of bed for dyspnea; palliative oxygen if needed

4. For DVT: use of antiembolic stockings applied before ambulation; expected anticoagulation medicine effects and side effects

5. Medicines, food and herbals that can affect anticoagulation including Vitamin E (greater than 1000–1500 units/day), theophylline, carbamazepine, phenytoin, Vitamin K (especially high in dark green vegetables)

6. For neutropenia: regular and frequent hand washing; plants, flowers not in direct proximity; support of family in encouraging visitors with colds, illness to visit when they are well

7. Review, rehearse with patient and family the steps to take if bleeding begins

G. Evaluate

1. Effectiveness of medical therapies

2. Patient compliance with anticoagulant therapy; for therapeutic PTT (partial thromboplastin time), PT (prothrombin time), INR (international normalized ratio)

3. Safety in ambulation

4. Patient/family understanding regarding disease process, safety, expected medicine effects and potential side effects

H. Revise plan according to findings from ongoing evaluations, changes in patient status or family needs

XVII. Hiccoughs

A. Definition: an involuntary contraction of the diaphragm, followed by rapid closure of the glottis

B. Possible Etiologies

1. Gastric distention: impaired gastric motility, excessive gas

2. Central nervous system: neoplasm, stroke, multiple sclerosis, ventriculoperitoneal shunts, arteriovenous malformations, hydrocephalus, lesions from head trauma

3. Peripheral nervous system: irritation of phrenic or vagus nerve

4. Tumors of the neck, lung, mediastinum

5. Chest surgery or trauma

6. Respiratory disorders: pulmonary edema, pneumonia, bronchitis, asthma, COPD

7. Gastrointestinal disorders: esophagitis or esophageal obstruction, gastritis, peptic ulcer disease, gastric cancer, pancreatitis, pancreatic cancer, bowel obstruction, cholelithiasis/cholecystitis

8. Renal/hepatic disorders

9. Metabolic disorders: uremia, hypocalcemia, hyponatremia

10. Infectious disease: sepsis, influenza, herpes zoster, malaria, tuberculosis

11. Pharmacologic agents: general anesthesia, IV corticosteroids, barbiturates, benzodiazepines, diazepam, chlordiazepoxide

12. Psychogenic: stress, excitement, grief reactions, anorexia, personality disorders

C.   Assess For

1.   Etiology of hiccoughs related to medical/psychological history and/or medication usage

2.   Associated signs and symptoms (underlying disease process, etc.)

3.   Severity and duration of current episode and previous episodes

4.   Relationship of hiccoughs to sleep: hiccoughs that stop during sleep suggest a psychogenic cause

5.   Patient/family concerns and knowledge: are the hiccoughs troublesome? Does anything help to alleviate hiccoughs?

D.   Diagnoses

1.   Alteration in comfort related to hiccoughs

2.   Risk for fluid/nutritional deficit related to dysphagia secondary to hiccoughs

3.   Risk for sleep pattern disturbance related to hiccoughs

4.   Patient/family knowledge deficit related to etiology and treatment of hiccoughs

E.   Planning and Intervention: etiology of hiccoughs can guide intervention plan (i.e., possible reversal of metabolic disorders)

1.   Non-pharmacologic interventions: before suggesting non-pharmacologic techniques, assure patient safety and do not suggest techniques that may be harmful, depending upon diagnosis

   a)   Nasopharyngeal stimulation

      i.   Swallowing one teaspoon of granulated sugar

      ii.   Lifting uvula with a spoon or cotton-tip applicator

      iii.   Gargling with water

      iv.   Biting on a lemon

      v.   Swallowing crushed ice

   b)   Interference with normal respiratory function

      i.   Induction of sneezing or coughing

      ii.   Re-breathing into paper bag

      iii.   Breath holding or hyperventilation

   c)   Etiology related to gastric distention

      i.   Nasogastric suction

      ii.   Gastric lavage

   d)   Complementary therapies

      i.   Hypnosis and/or behavior modification

      ii.   Acupuncture

   e)   Distraction

2. Pharmacologic Therapies

    a) If etiology is related to gastric distention

        i. Simethicone before or after meals

        ii. Metoclopramide alone or with simethicone before meals

    b) Peppermint oil relaxes lower esophageal sphincter and is useful for hiccoughs related to esophageal disorders; has opposing action with metoclopramide

    c) Baclofen (5–10 mg po tid, prn) if simethicone and metoclopramide fail

    d) Calcium channel blockers, e.g., NIFEdipine

    e) Chlorpromazine 25–50 mg tid effective for uremic etiology, but useful in other etiologies as well; postural hypotension a significant side effect, especially when used IV

    f) Anticonvulsants: carbamazepine, phenytoin, and valproic acid

    g) Nebulized lidocaine (3 ml of injectable 2% nebulized lidocaine in a standard small-particle nebulizer)

3. Invasive Techniques

    a) Phrenic nerve interruption with bupivacaine or surgery

    b) Pacing electrodes for direct phrenic nerve or diaphragmatic stimulation

F. Patient/Family Education

1. Explain etiology and instruct in ways to treat

2. Explain appropriate, safe non-pharmacological techniques that are realistic for individual patient

3. Expected medication effects and side effects

4. Post-surgical care, if indicated

G. Evaluate

1. Effectiveness of non-pharmacological techniques and/or medication

2. Control of hiccoughs

3. Patient/family understanding of regimen

H. Revise plan according to findings from ongoing evaluations, changes in patient status or family needs

XVIII. Impaired Mobility, Fatigue, Lethargy, Weakness

A. **Definitions**

1. Impaired mobility: a loss or abnormality of function due to physiological, anatomical, psychological or fatigue factors

2. Fatigue: a subjective sense of exhaustion with decreased motivation, ability to do activities and a decreased capacity for physical or mental activity[12]

3. Lethargy: advanced fatigue

4. Weakness: a subjective term to indicate a lack of strength as compared to what patient feels is normal

B. **Potential Etiologies**

1. Disease process

   a) Sudden onset of weakness or impaired mobility: consider neurologic deficit, e.g., spinal cord compression or other CNS tumor effects; sudden generalized weakness may be adrenal failure or septicemia

   b) Chronic disease: chronic obstructive pulmonary disease (COPD), congestive heart failure (CHF)

   c) Tumor infiltration of bone marrow

   d) Liver disease with coagulopathy

   e) Hypothyroidism; adrenal or hormonal insufficiencies (including chemical and hormonal response to tumor)

   f) Uremia: related to kidney failure, tumor, or use of nephrotoxic drugs

   g) Metabolic: hypercalcemia from metastatic disease, parathyroid disease

2. Uncontrolled pain or other symptoms, anemia, blood loss

3. Some medications or therapies may contribute to lethargy, weakness: beta blockers, antihistamines, benzodiazepines, phenothiazines, zidovudine (AZT®), myelosuppressive chemotherapy, radiation therapy

4. Nutritional deficiencies

   a) Decreased iron, B-12, folate

   b) Anorexia, nausea, vomiting, weight loss

   c) GI malabsorption

5. Infectious processes

   a) AIDS-related infections

   b) Pneumonia

   c) Urinary tract infections

6. Emotional factors: depression, anxiety, sleep disturbance, psychological or spiritual distress, family distress

7. Environmental factors: multiple sensory stimuli (noise, lights, odors)

C.   Assess for Etiology, which will determine intervention plan

1. Thorough history

   a) Onset, history of or change in functional status

   b) Patient's own description of fatigue, weakness: does it relate to activity? Is it constant? Intermittent?

   c) Effect of fatigue, weakness and lethargy on quality of life using a number scale of 1 (no fatigue) to 10 (extreme fatigue)[12]

   d) Patient's place on disease trajectory of end-stage or terminal illness

2. Symptom management: review adequacy of pain control and management of other debilitating symptoms (including nausea, vomiting, dyspnea, anxiety, depression)

3. Current medications for appropriate use and dose for patient's current weight

4. Psychosocial factors

   a) Sleep, rest disturbance

   b) Depression, anxiety component

   c) Unresolved psychological or spiritual issues or distress

5. Family, caregiver perceptions and impact of patient's fatigue; understanding of disease process

6. Infectious or disease process

7. Dyspnea if anemic

D.   Potential Diagnoses

1. Activity alteration from fatigue due to (etiology)

2. Self-care deficit related to activity intolerance

3. Risk for altered nutritional, functional status due to activity disturbance

4. Patient/family knowledge deficit of non-pharmacologic interventions, expected medication effects, side effects

5. Impaired physical mobility related to [injury, potential for injury, pain]

6. Alteration in perceived quality of life from fatigue

7. Altered self-image and role disturbance related to change in functional abilities and endurance

E. Planning and Interventions: etiology of fatigue, impaired mobility, lethargy and weakness will determine intervention plan

1. Patient's place on disease trajectory for end-stage or terminal illness, wishes and advance directives will influence treatment decisions

2. Treat specific underlying causes as appropriate

   a) If anemia: based on classification of anemia, consider treatment of cause

   b) If endocrine disorder: determine appropriate therapy

   c) If medication-induced (iatrogenic)

      i. Consider tapering or discontinuing medicine

      ii. If opioid induced, fatigue may resolve when patient develops tolerance (usually 48–72 hours after dose increase)

      iii. If opioid induced lethargy continues and other etiologies have been ruled out and is unacceptable to the patient/family, consider adding methylphenidate 5 mg po in the A.M. and at noon to combat sedation and to improve appetite and mood.[13] Titrate if not effective

3. Non-pharmacologic interventions

   a) Balance activities with rest

   b) Hospital bed and other equipment as needed to decrease fatigue from exertion

   c) Set realistic goals for ADLs and other activities

   d) Exercise, physical and occupational therapy as indicated, if tolerated

   e) Increase team services for personal care as needed

F. Patient/Family Education

1. Instruct regarding balancing activities and rest

2. Set activity priorities: e.g., a bedside commode may help patient to conserve the energy used walking to the bathroom for other activities

3. Expected medication effects and potential side effects especially as they may contribute to fatigue or sedation

4. Educate family of hospice patient in terminal phase regarding end-stage disease process and encourage setting of realistic expectations

5. For the palliative care patient who is not in terminal phase of disease process, discourage prolonged bedrest or excessive inactivity explaining possible adverse physical (deep vein thrombosis [DVT], pulmonary embolism [PE], pneumonia, increased weakness) and emotional (depression, decreased motivation, social isolation) effects

G. Evaluate

1. Effectiveness of interventions and ability of the caregivers to provide care

2. Improvement in activity tolerance

3. Patient for signs of disease progression

4. Patient/family understanding, coping with ongoing fatigue, balancing activities, prioritizing to accomplish essential or preferred activities

5. Further adjustments in team visit frequency to assist in personal care as needed

H. Revise plan according to findings from ongoing evaluations, changes in patient status or family needs

XIX. Increased Intracranial Pressure (ICP)

A. Definition: increase in the pressure within the cranial cavity due to increased volume of fluid or mass

B. Possible Etiologies

1 Space occupying tumors, metastatic lesions with surrounding edema

2. Intracranial hemorrhage

3. Inflammatory process: abscess, encephalitis, meningitis

4. Obstruction of CSF flow

C. Assess For

1. Sudden unanticipated changes in patient condition with signs of increased ICP: new headache, vomiting, changed respiratory pattern, decreased motor function, lethargy to altered mental status, increased restlessness, agitation, blurred vision

2. Documentation of possible etiologies of increased ICP in past medical history

3. Patient and family anxiety, ability to cope with changes in condition; knowledge and/or understanding of presenting changes, disease process, treatment options

D. Potential Diagnoses

1. Altered mental status due to increased ICP

2. Cerebral alteration related to increased ICP

3. Patient and family knowledge deficit related to: disease process, current symptom changes, coping strategies

E. Planning and Interventions

1. Treat underlying etiology if appropriate

2. Steroids to reduce edema/inflammation

3. Anticonvulsant if seizure activity

4. Palliative radiotherapy when appropriate

5. Analgesia for headache

    a) Keep in mind that opioids can mildly increase ICP due to vasodilatation effects and mild respiratory depression

    b) Tramadol should not be used in increased ICP as it may lower seizure threshold[14]

6. Non-pharmacologic measures: head of bed 45–60 degrees, darkened room, reduce external stimuli in environment, calm presence

F. Patient/Family Education

1. Reassurance and instruction regarding possible cause for changes in patient condition

2. Review goals of therapy to reduce intracranial pressure symptoms and increase patient comfort and safety

3. Preparation for changes that may indicate advancement of disease and decline of patient condition; support of family/caregiver goals, needs

4. Consider transfer of home hospice patient to inpatient hospice facility or palliative care facility bed if management is beyond physical, emotional capacity of family or caregiver

G. Evaluate

1. Effectiveness of medications, patient comfort and relief, reduction of increased ICP symptoms

2. Patient/family understanding, coping, anxiety related to current symptoms, plan

H. Revise plan according to findings from ongoing evaluations, changes in patient status or family needs

XX. Myoclonus

A. Definition: twitching or brief spasm of a muscle or muscle group

B. Possible Etiologies

1. High dose opioid therapy

2. Metabolic derangement, e.g., uremia

3. Inflammatory or degenerative CNS diseases, e.g., Creutzfeldt-Jakob, subacute sclerosing panencephalitis, end-stage Alzheimer's

4. Hypercalcemia from osteoblastic activity of bone metastases

C. Assess For

1. Onset, duration of myoclonus and its impact on patient and patient functional status

2. Interruption of sleep, rest

3. Patient/family anxiety related to myoclonic jerking

4. Patient/family understanding of disease process, medication effects and side effects

5. Potential etiology which will direct intervention plan

    a) If opioid-induced, evaluate adjuvant use that would allow for pain to be managed using a reduced opioid dose or rotate opioids. Dose can often be decreased because of incomplete cross tolerance

    b) If hypercalcemia, evaluate patient's place on the disease trajectory

6. Patient safety if ambulatory or if bed bound due to uncontrolled muscular jerking movements

D. Potential Diagnoses

1. Alteration in metabolic status related to uremia, hypercalcemia, etc.

2. Alteration in functional status due to impairment of neuro-musculoskeletal system

3. Disturbance of sleep and rest pattern due to myoclonus

4. Patient/family knowledge deficit regarding: medication effects, disease process, safety precautions

E. Planning and Intervention: Etiology of myoclonus will direct intervention plan

1. Non-pharmacologic adjunct therapies including local heat, gentle massage, relaxation

2. If hypercalcemia etiology

    a) In palliative care, may consider pamidronate or zoledronic q 3–4 weeks to decrease serum calcium

    b) In hospice, supplementary hydration (IV or PO) may decrease serum calcium and relieve symptoms

3. If opioid-induced, consider adjuvant medicines for the specific type of pain (neuropathic or bone) at the most appropriate dose that may allow reduction in opioid dose or rotate opioids

4. If unable to treat underlying metabolic or degenerative disorder because of advanced stage of disease, patient/family wishes, treat symptoms with clonazepam, valproic acid

5. Occasionally muscle relaxants provide benefit

    a) Diazepam

    b) Baclofen

    c) Cyclobenzaprine

        i. Cyclobenzaprine should be used cautiously in elderly or debilitated patients and considered a second line to baclofen

        ii. Increases side effects of other medications often taken by the elderly and has side effects that can contribute to conditions often already present such as CHF, glaucoma, etc.

6. If night cramps only, quinine sulfate at bedtime

F. **Patient/Family Education**

1. Discuss possible etiologies and recommended interventions

2. Expected medication effects and potential side effects

3. Non-pharmacologic methods of intervention: heat, gentle massage, relaxation to decrease anxiety

G. **Evaluate for effectiveness of interventions, specifically**

1. Decrease in or resolution of myoclonus

2. Maintenance of effective pain control

3. Patient/family understanding of instructions, recommendations

4. Patient safety

H. **Revise plan according to findings from ongoing evaluations, changes in patient status or family needs**

XXI. Nausea and Vomiting

A. **Definitions**

1. Nausea is a subjectively perceived, stomach discomfort ranging from stomach awareness to the conscious recognition of the need to vomit

2. Vomiting is the expelling of stomach contents through the mouth

B. **Possible Etiologies[3,7,15]**

1. Fluid and electrolyte imbalances (hypercalcemia, hyponatremia, uremia, dehydration)

2. Gastrointestinal disorders (pressure due to tumor, organomegaly; distention; ascites; esophageal, gastrointestinal, and hepatic malignancies; constipation; bowel obstruction; GI stasis)

3. Other physiologic disorders (oral thrush; cough; pain; high fever)

4. Neurologic disorders (primary and metastatic CNS tumors, increased intracranial pressure)

5. Renal failure

6. Vestibular (tumors and bone metastases at skull base; motion sickness)

7. Chemical (radiation, medications such as chemotherapy, antibiotics, aspirin, iron, steroids, digoxin, expectorants, NSAIDs, opioids, theophylline)

8. Psychogenic (anxiety; anticipatory nausea and vomiting; fear)

9. Adverse response to certain foods especially high fat content

10. Adverse response to certain drugs e.g., increase in opioids

C. **Assess For**

1. History of the onset of nausea and vomiting and concomitant symptoms i.e., heartburn, constipation, excessive thirst and other symptoms that can indicate etiology

2. Pattern of nausea: when does nausea occur? Are there contributing factors?

3. If possible, assess vomitus for volume, color, odor, presence of blood (vomitus with fecal odor or fecal material indicates possible bowel obstruction; coffee ground emesis indicates old blood, whereas fresh blood indicates current hemorrhage)

4. Abdominal assessment: pain or cramps, bowel sounds, distention

5. Oropharynx for infection (thrush) or presence of tenacious sputum

6. Neurologic signs of increased intracranial pressure

7. Other factors that could trigger nausea response: malodorous wounds, pain, fear, anxiety

D. **Potential Diagnoses**

1. Nausea related to metabolic disorders, tumor pressure, drug therapies, neurosensory disorders, or anxiety

2. Risk for fluid volume deficit related to nausea and vomiting

3. Risk for altered nutrition due to intake less than body requirements related to inability to eat or keep food down secondary to nausea and vomiting

4. Patient/family knowledge deficit related to etiology and treatment of nausea and vomiting

E. **Planning and Intervention: Etiology of nausea and vomiting may guide interventions**

1. Modify diet to decrease nausea

    a) Bland foods that patient enjoys, e.g., baked potatoes, soft fruits, yogurt, soft drinks, crackers or dry toast, clear liquids such as Popsicles®, JELL-O®, sports drinks, foods without aggressive odors or those that produce gas

    b) Cold or room temperature foods are often better tolerated than warm foods due to less odor

    c) Serve small, frequent meals

    d) Avoid fatty, greasy, spicy or very sweet foods

2. Correct reversible causes of nausea, including cough, hypercalcemia, increased intracranial pressure

3. Stop/hold suspected medication and obtain serum levels (digoxin, theophylline) as appropriate depending on patient's goal

4. Keep the patient cool; place a fan in the room or open a window to circulate air

5. Keep patient's head elevated

6. Medication regimen (see Table 3) should be prescribed according to etiology of nausea[3,16]

    a) A prokinetic agent (metoclopramide) can be used for delayed gastric emptying (do not use in bowel obstruction)

    b) Butyrophenones, i.e., haloperidol or droperidol (Inapsine®)for opioid-induced nausea (nausea related to opioid initiation generally resolves within one week)

    c) An antihistamine (meclizine, dimenhyDRINATE) can be used for bowel obstruction or other visceral irritation (liver metastases, constipation, etc.), disturbances in the vestibular system (vertigo, motion sickness), pharyngeal stimulation (tenacious sputum, oral thrush), or increased intracranial pressure (which can also be treated with a glucocorticoid such as dexamethasone)

    d) Anticholinergics (scopolamine patches, hydroxyzine) are used primarily for increased intracranial pressure and vestibular disturbances

    e) Nausea related to disturbances in the chemoreceptor trigger zone (CTZ) (usually due to metabolic disorders, medications, and toxins produced from GI tumors, infection, poisoning, etc.), can be treated by discontinuing offending medication if possible, and utilizing drugs which act on the CTZ (haloperidol, metoclopramide, phenothiazines)

    f) Nausea related to emetogenic chemotherapy can be treated with 5-HT$_3$ serotonin receptor antagonists (ondansetron, granisetron)

    g) Nausea related to anxiety and fear can be treated with antihistamines or anticholinergics

7. Oral hygiene before and after meals

F. Patient/Family Education

1. Explain etiology and treatment course of nausea and vomiting

2. Explain effects of medication and possible side effects

3. Explain non-pharmacologic measures to treat nausea and vomiting, including diet, oral hygiene, etc.

G. Evaluate

1. Effectiveness of interventions and patient/family teaching (are patient/family satisfied with outcome?)

2. Medication effectiveness and presence of side effects

3. Patient/family understanding of treatment measures

H. Revise plan according to findings from ongoing evaluations, changes in patient status or family needs

Table 3: Management of Nausea/Vomiting[a]

Syndrome Pathway(s)[b]	Causes	Clinical Features	Antiemetic Management	Adjuvant
S Gastric stasis and gastric outflow obstruction **P** Vomiting center, GI tract	Anticholinergic drugs, autonomic failure, ascites, hepatomegaly, tumor infiltration, peptic ulcer, gastritis	Epigastric fullness and discomfort. Early satiety. Flatulence, hiccup, acid reflux and gastric regurgitation. Large volume emesis which may contain undigested food. Nausea often relieved by vomiting	Prokinetic Metoclopramide 10–20 mg tid po 40–80 mg sub-Q infusion/24 hours	Dietary advice. Paracentesis for ascites. Simethicone for flatulence. Steroid therapy may be used to improve the dysfunction induced by tumor infiltration of nerve plexuses. For total obstruction a venting gastrostomy or surgical bypass may be considered. H_2 blocker or proton pump inhibitor. Review drug regimen.
S Stretch/ irritation of visceral and GI serosa **P** Vomiting center, GI tract	Liver metastases, ureteric obstruction, tumor, constipation, bowel obstruction, lymph nodes	Pain is often a feature. Colic. Altered bowel habits. Nausea. Vomiting of fecal fluid in obstruction.	Antihistamine *DiphenhydrAMINE* 25–50 mg tid or qid po/IM/IV *Promethazine* 12.5–25 mg tid or qid po/IM/IV/PR *Hydroxyzine* 25–100 mg tid or qid po/IM	Relieve the cause, e.g., constipation with stimulant laxatives and enemas as required. Steroid therapy for the reduction of peri-tumor edema

[a]Adapted with permission from: Campbell, T. & Hately, J. (2000). The management of nausea and vomiting in advanced cancer. *International Journal of Palliative Nursing, 6*(1): pp. 18–20, 22–25.

[b]Editor's Note: **S** = Syndrome, **P** = Pathway(s).

Table 3: Management of Nausea/Vomiting (cont)

Syndrome Pathway(s)	Causes	Clinical Features	Antiemetic Management	Adjuvant
S Raised intracranial pressure/ meningism **P** Vomiting center	Cerebral tumor, intracranial tumor, intracranial bleeding, infiltration of meninges by tumor, skull metastases, cerebral infection	Neurological signs, e.g. cyclovir, drowsiness, dizziness, headache, nausea and/or vomiting, vomiting may be projectile in nature	Antihistamine *Diphenhydramine* 25–50 mg tid or qid po/IM/IV *Promethazine* 12.5–25 mg tid or qid po/IM/IV/PR *Hydroxyzine* 25–100 mg tid or qid po/IM Dexamethasone Anticholinergic *Scopolamine Transdermal patch* q 3 days	High dose steroids may reduce cerebral edema and/or tumor mass
S Pharyngeal stimulation **P** Vomiting center	Tenacious sputum not easily expectorated, infection *(Candida)*	Retching	Antihistamine *Diphenhydramine* 25–50 mg tid or qid po/IM/IV *Promethazine* 12.5–25 mg tid or qid po/IM/IV/PR *Hydroxyzine* 25–100 mg tid or qid po/IM	Treat the cause. Saline nebulizers. Antibiotics. Antifungal therapy.
S Esophageal obstruction **P** Vomiting center	Tumor, odynophagia (painful swallowing), functional dysphagia, *Candida*	Regurgitation, dysphagia	Anticholinergic Will help to reduce saliva and secretions *Scopolamine Transdermal patch* q 3 days	Radiotherapy, brachiotherapy, laser therapy, high dose steroids, self-expanding stent, Celestin or Atkinson tube, Surgery (not for patients with metastatic spread)
S Anxiety **P** Vomiting center	Psychological and emotional distress, anticipatory emesis associated with chemotherapy	Nausea, waves of nausea and vomiting, distraction may relieve symptoms	Antihistamine or Anticholinergics if required	Address the anxiety with psychological techniques. Relaxation. Benzodiazepines. Ensure adequate pain control.

XXII. Paresthesia and Neuropathy

A. Definitions

1. Paresthesia: a sensation of numbness, prickling or tingling; heightened sensitivity

2. Neuropathy: any disease of the nerves; may include sensory loss, muscle weakness and atrophy and decreased deep tendon reflexes

B. Possible Etiologies

1. Central and peripheral nerve lesions

2. Direct damage to peripheral and autonomic nerves

3. Metabolic and vascular changes of diabetes mellitus

4. Chemical or drug-induced: e.g., chemotherapy, isoniazid, alcohol

5. Amputation, AIDS, vitamin B_{12} deficiency

6. Tumor invasion with pressure on nerves or plexuses

7. Spinal cord compression (considered an oncologic emergency)

C. Assess For

1. Sudden loss of sensation, motor function of lower extremities with or without loss of bladder or bowel control; **MAY INDICATE SPINAL CORD COMPRESSION WHICH IS A MEDICAL EMERGENCY.** Most common signs of pending cord compression are escalating back pain with or without bladder changes and before lower extremity weakness, worse when lying down, improved when standing. Amount of neurological deficit patient presents with is usually amount left with following treatment, therefore early recognition is imperative

2. Location and degree of numbness: patient's subjective descriptions of pain or sensation assist in determining etiology

3. Patient's course in the diseases process/trajectory for assistance in intervention planning

4. Patient safety in ambulation, ADLs

5. Patient/family understanding of cause of sudden change in sensation or motor function, need for safety in ambulation/ADLs, understanding of treatment options

D. Potential Diagnoses

1. Alteration in comfort related to peripheral sensory and neuropathic changes

2. Safety risk related to alteration in sensation

3. Patient/family knowledge deficit related to safety needs, medication effects, treatment options

4. Compromised patient/family coping related to uncontrolled pain

E. **Planning and Intervention: determining patient's course in disease process, trajectory will facilitate planning in the event of spinal cord compression**

1. If patient is in advanced stage of disease (weak, bed bound, poor nutritional status), symptom management may be appropriate option, i.e., steroids to decrease edema around cord; neuroleptic analgesia, opioids

2. If patient is ambulatory, active and able to participate in self-care, palliative radiotherapy and steroids may provide significant benefit for quality of life

3. Tricyclic antidepressants (TCAs) are appropriate adjuvant analgesics to opioids for neuropathic pain (see Chapter IV, Section III. A. 1. d.)

    a) Titrate dose every few days based upon the patient's response

    b) Therapeutic levels achieved in 3–7 days

4. Anticonvulsants can be considered for neuropathic pain:

    a) If gabapentin: start low (e.g. 200–300 mg qHS). Dose can be titrated to 3600 mg daily maximum (in divided doses) for therapeutic effect

    b) If carbamazepine or phenytoin: monitor for effect and for drug interaction (monitor serum levels, CBC)

5. Appropriate bowel regimen if patient has decreased activity, is bed bound or has lost sensation in rectum

6. Foley catheter for urinary retention

7. Condom or Foley catheter for urinary incontinence if this causes skin irritation, patient anxiety and if patient/caregiver agree

8. Increase assistance with ADLs in home as indicated for patient personal needs and safety

F. **Patient/Family Education**

1. Expected medication effects and possible side effects

    a) Continue TCAs regularly

        i. It takes 3–7 days to become therapeutic for neuropathic pain

        ii. Give at night, which might aid in sleeping and reduce daytime sedation

    b) Prepare patient/family to expect that gabapentin may cause sedation when initiated or dose increased

    c) Carbamazepine may cause dizziness, drowsiness, anorexia and nausea

    d) Phenytoin may cause ataxia, diplopia, dizziness, drowsiness

2. Safety needs when ambulating related to decreased sensation, motor ability and medication effects

G. **Evaluate for effectiveness of interventions, specifically**

    1. Compliance with medication regimen

    2. Effectiveness of medication and any side effects

    3. Return of sensation, function

    4. Safety needs/issues

H. **Revise plan according to findings from ongoing evaluations, changes in patient status or family needs**

XXIII. Seizures

A. **Definitions: usually intermittent tonic, clonic movements; convulsions caused by a large number of neurons discharging abnormally[17]**

    1. Primary (generalized) involving large parts of the brain and including grand mal and petit mal types

    2. Focal (partial) involving specific regions of the brain with symptoms reflecting the location of the disturbance

B. **Possible Etiologies[17]**

    1. Brain infarct, primary brain tumor or brain metastases, cerebral abscess, brain infection in HIV and AIDS

    2. Increased intracranial pressure (may be associated with SIADH in some cancer patients)

    3. Pre-existing seizure disorder

    4. Medications (metabolites from normeperidine and propoxyphene) and their preservatives (sodium bisulfite); medications that lower seizure threshold include phenothiazines, butyrophenones, tricyclic antidepressants

    5. Infection, stroke, hemorrhage, oxygen deprivation, paraneoplastic syndromes

    6. Metabolic instability (hyponatremia, hypercalcemia, hypomagnesemia, hypoxemia, hypoglycemia)

    7. Drug toxicity, drug withdrawal

C. **Assess For**

    1. Acutely seizing patient: intervene with first intervention below

    2. Underlying etiology reviewing medical history, disease process, current medications, history of trauma or recent fall, differentiate from myoclonus

    3. Question patient and/or family to determine onset and type of seizure, presence of aura, headache, nausea and projectile vomiting

    4. Drug levels if previously taking anticonvulsants; EEG may be warranted

    5. Patient/family coping with seizure activity, their understanding of patient protection/safety during seizure, medication effects and side effects

D.   Potential Diagnoses

1.   Safety precautions (e.g., risk for falls) for seizures from: etiology

2.   Potential risk for medication toxicity or withdrawal side effects

   a)   Dexamethasone is commonly given to those with seizure disorder; interaction between this drug and phenytoin is problematic, monitor phenytoin levels as appropriate

   b)   Steroids must not be suddenly stopped—seizures may occur

3.   Metabolic impairment related to: hyponatremia, hypercalcemia, hypomagnesemia, hypoxia, hypoglycemia

4.   Patient/family knowledge deficit related to: etiology, disease process, medication effects/side effects, safety

E.   Planning and Intervention

1.   For actively seizing patient

   a)   Assess airway, breathing, circulation and ensure adequate airway

   b)   Protect patient from harm and ensure safety

   c)   Model calm demeanor

   d)   Medical therapy may include

      i.   IV lorazepam (drug of choice)

      ii.   Diazepam enema, IV diazepam

      iii. Fosphenytoin (Cerebyx®) IV

      iv.   Initiation of phenytoin, carbamazepine, valproic acid or phenobarbital[20]

2.   Determine potentially treatable etiologies

   a)   Hypoglycemia: glucose PO/IV or glucagon SQ as indicated

   b)   Hyponatremia: fluid restriction, IV NaCl, adjustment of diuretics

   c)   Hypercalcemia: increase fluids PO/IV, pamidronate may be appropriate depending on disease trajectory

   d)   Hypoxemia: supplemental O_2; further evaluation of this etiology

   e)   Hypomagnesemia: supplemental magnesium

   f)   Infectious process (cerebral abscess, encephalitis, meningitis): antibiotics as indicated and according to patient's place on disease trajectory and advance directives

   g)   Substance abuse: support withdrawal, consult substance withdrawal specialist

F. Patient/Family Education

    1. Anticipate potential for seizure activity and prepare family for patient safety, preemptive interventions, whom to call

    2. Calmly rehearse, review caregiver interventions

    3. Expected medication effects and potential side effects

G. Evaluate

    1. Effectiveness of seizure management interventions

    2. Family preparedness and coping

    3. Patient safety

    4. Medication effects and side effects

    5. Blood draws to monitor levels of medications such as phenytoin

        a) Phenytoin has a narrow therapeutic range, and drug interactions may lead to alterations in its plasma concentration

H. Revise plan according to findings from ongoing evaluations, changes in patient status or family needs

XXIV. Urinary Incontinence/Retention[18]

A. Definition: the inability to control urination

B. Possible Etiologies

    1. Urge incontinence: urge to void sensed, but cannot control urine flow long enough to reach toilet

        a) Due to bladder irritation such as infection, tumor, radiation, or chemotherapy

        b) Nervous system damage: spinal cord lesions (neurogenic bladder), stroke, multiple sclerosis, Parkinson's, Alzheimer's

        c) Decreased mobility or difficulty reaching the toilet in time

    2. Stress incontinence: leakage of urine when intra-abdominal pressure is raised

        a) Damage or dysfunction of bladder sphincter due to

            i. Tumor infiltration in GU system or CNS or spinal cord lesions

            ii. Multiparity or post-menopausal changes in women

    3. Overflow incontinence: bladder unable to empty normally

        a) Bladder outlet obstruction due to fecal mass, tumor, calculi, prostatic hypertrophy

        b) Detrusor muscle failure due to anticholinergic drugs, CNS lesions, or debility and confusion

4. Functional incontinence: an involuntary or unpredictable passage of urine with no impairment of the GU tract

   a) Cognitive dysfunction: depression leading to self-neglect, confusion, excessive sedation

   b) Mobility or functional problems: Immobility, unable to undress, inaccessible toilet facilities, final stage of illness

5. Many drugs can lead to any of the aforementioned urinary incontinence problems

   a) Diuretics increase volume and frequency

   b) Sedatives decrease awareness of need to void, as well as decrease bladder contraction and outlet resistance

   c) Anticholinergics decrease bladder contraction

   d) Antiparkinsonian drugs increase outlet resistance

6. Metabolic disorders: hypercalcemia

7. Atonic bladder: no awareness of bladder fullness or urgency

   a) Diabetic neuropathy

   b) Spinal cord lesions or cord compression

   c) Neurologic dysfunction

8. Fistula

C. **Assess For**

1. History, including nature and duration of symptoms, medications, recent treatments for cancer

2. Physical exam: bladder distention, perineal swelling, fecal impaction, simple neurologic exam (including sensation and sensorimotor deficits), signs of hypercalcemia, functional assessment (mobility, able to dress/undress self, presence of aphasia or dysphasia), skin assessment

3. Urge incontinence: nocturia, frequency with urination

4. Stress incontinence: leakage of urine upon laughing, coughing, sneezing, lifting or bending

5. Overflow incontinence: bladder distention, discomfort, urgency, continual dribbling and only voiding small amounts, large residual urine after voiding, fecal impaction

6. Functional incontinence: mobility, ability to perform ADLs, cognitive level, depression

D. **Diagnoses**

1. Altered urinary elimination related to anatomic dysfunction or obstruction, medications, or metabolic disorder

2. Urinary incontinence, urge, related to bladder irritation, sensory-motor disorder, or decreased mobility

3. Urinary incontinence, stress, related to decrease in bladder or sphincter support

4. Urinary incontinence, functional, related to cognitive dysfunction or mobility problems

5. Risk for impaired skin integrity related to urinary incontinence

6. Patient/family knowledge deficit related to etiology and management of urinary incontinence

7. Patient/family anxiety related to urinary incontinence

8. Risk for falls trying to get to the bathroom

E. Planning and Intervention

1. Review medications and discontinue those that may be causing incontinence (if appropriate). Medications that can cause urinary incontinence include opioids, sedatives, antidepressants, antipsycotics, antiparkinsonian drugs and alpha-aderdergic blocking agents[18]

2. If appropriate, establish a regular voiding schedule (i.e., every 2 hours)

3. Alter environment to make toileting easier (i.e., move patient closer to toilet, or utilize a bedside commode, urinal, or bedpan, assuring modesty and dignity is maintained)

4. Decrease fluid intake at night, and limit intake of food/fluids containing caffeine or alcohol

5. If fecal impaction is present, disimpact and teach bowel regime to patient and family to avoid further problems

6. Consider catheterizing, either indwelling or external

7. Utilize incontinence supplies, such as pads, briefs, etc.

8. Teach patient and family hygiene and skin care measures

9. Urge incontinence: oxybutynin (Ditropan®) or tolterodine (Detrol®) (long acting products preferred). Antibiotics for UTI, urinary tract analgesics such as phenazopyridine (Pyridium®) for pain, imipramine for neurogenic bladder[18]

10. Stress incontinence: teach pelvic floor muscle exercises (PFME) and voiding schedule, pessary or penile clamp, imipramine at bedtime for anticholinergic effect

11. Overflow incontinence: discontinue anticholinergic medications, if possible; disimpact if necessary; cholinergic drug such as bethanechol (Urecholine®); indwelling catheterization if obstruction persists

12. Functional incontinence: interventions rely on cause of incontinence; indwelling catheter may be only choice

13. Incontinence related to fistulas is treated by establishing voiding schedules, catheterization, and, if indicated, urinary diversion (if life expectancy is not short)

F. Patient/Family Education

1. Expected medication effects and potential side effects

2. Demonstrate correct hygiene and skin care techniques to prevent skin breakdown

3. Explain correct catheter care and signs of catheter malfunction

4. Explain safety measures if altering environment for ease in toileting (i.e., have patient call for assistance, voiding schedules, assuring clear path to bathroom)

5. Explain signs and symptoms of urinary tract infection (UTI)

G. Evaluate

1. Effectiveness of interventions (are patient/family satisfied with outcome?)

2. Skin integrity

3. Medication effects and side effects

4. Patient safety

H. Revise plan according to findings from ongoing evaluations, changes in patient/family needs

CITED REFERENCES

1. Bergstrom N, et al., *Pressure Ulcer Treatment: Clinical Practice Guideline. Quick Reference Guide for Clinicians, No. 15*. Rockville, MD: U.S. Department of Health and Human Services, Public Health Service, Agency for Health Care Policy and Research; 1994.

2. Dahlin CM, Goldsmith T. Dysphagia, dry mouth, & hiccups. In: Ferrell BR, Coyle N. eds. *Textbook of Palliative Nursing*. New York, NY: Oxford University Press; 2001:122–138.

3. Waller A, Caroline NL. *Handbook of Palliative Care in Cancer*. 2nd ed. Boston, MA: Butterworth-Heinemann; 2000.

4. Rhiner M, Slatkin NE. Pruritus, fever, and sweats, In: Ferrell BR, Coyle N. Eds. *Textbook of Palliative Nursing*. New York, NY: Oxford University Press; 2001:245–261.

5. Kuebler KK, English N, Heidrich DE. Delirium, confusion, agitation, and restlessness, In: Ferrell BR, Coyle N. Eds. *Textbook of Palliative Nursing*. New York, NY: Oxford University Press; 2001:290–308.

6. Collins CA. Ascites. *Clinical Journal of Oncology Nursing,* 2001;5(1):43–44.

7. Kemp C. *Terminal Illness: A Guide to Nursing Care*. 2nd ed. Philadelphia, PA: Lippincott; 1999.

8. Letizia M, Norton E. Successful management of malignant bowel obstruction. *Journal of Hospice and Palliative Nursing*. 2002:5(3):152–158.

9. Kazanowski MK. Symptom management in palliative care. In: Matzo ML, Sherman DW, eds. *Palliative Care Nursing: Quality Care to the End of Life*. New York, NY: Springer Publishing; 2001:327–361.

10. Dudgeon D. Dyspnea, death rattle, and cough. In: Ferrell BR, Coyle N. Eds. *Textbook of Palliative Nursing*. New York, NY: Oxford University Press; 2001:164–174.

11. Runyan BA. Management of adult patients with ascites due to cirrhosis. *AASLD Practice Guideline*. Available at http://www.ikp.unibe.ch/lab2/aasldascites2004.pdf. Accessed March 1, 2005.

12. Dean GE, Anderson PR. Fatigue. In: Ferrell BR, Coyle N. Eds. *Textbook of Palliative Nursing*. New York, NY: Oxford University Press; 2001:91–100.

13. Chochinov HM, and Breitbart W. *Handbook of Psychiatry and Palliative Care*. New York, NY: Oxford University Press; 2000.

14. McCaffery M, Pasero C. *Pain: Clinical Manual*. St. Louis, MO: Mosby; 1999.

15. Miller K, Miller M. Managing common gastrointestinal symptoms at the end of life. *Journal of Hospice and Palliative Nursing*. 2002:4(1):34–42.

16. Campbell T, Hately J. The management of nausea and vomiting in advanced cancer. *International Journal of Palliative Nursing*. 2000;6(1): 18–20, 22–25.

17. Paice JA. Neurological disturbances, In: Ferrell BR, Coyle N. eds. *Textbook of Palliative Nursing*. New York, NY: Oxford University Press; 2001;262–268.

18. Gray M, Campbell FG. Urinary tract disorders In: Ferrell BR, Coyle N. Eds. *Textbook of Palliative Nursing*. New York, NY: Oxford University Press; 2001:175–191.

ADDITIONAL REFERENCES AND RESOURCES

Ersek M. Artificial nutrition and hydration: clinical issues. *Journal of Hospice and Palliative Nursing.* 2002:5(4):221–230.

Evans BD. Improving palliative care in the nursing home: from a dementia perspective. *Journal of Hospice and Palliative Nursing.* 2002:4(2):91–99.

Jablonski A, Wyatt GK. A model for identifying barriers to effective symptom management at the end of life. *Journal of Hospice and Palliative Nursing.* 2002:23–36.

Kolcaba K, Dowd T, Steiner R, Mitzer A. Efficacy of hand massage for enhancing the comfort of hospice patients. *Journal of Hospice and Palliative Nursing.* 2002:6(2):91–102.

Lentz J. Daily baths: torment or comfort at end of life. *Journal of Hospice and Palliative Nursing.* 2002:5(1):34–39.

Sander R. Promoting urinary continence in residential care. *Nursing Standard.* 2000;14(13):49–54.

Smith SA, ed. *Hospice and Palliative Nurses Association Monograph: Treatment of End-Stage Non-Cancer Diagnoses.* Dubuque, IA: Kendall/Hunt Publishing; 2001.

Panke JA, Volicer L. Caring for persons with dementia: a palliative approach. *Journal of Hospice and Palliative Nursing.* 2002:4(3):143–149.

Wrede-Seaman L. *Symptom Management Algorithms for Palliative Care.* Yakima, WA: Intellicard; 1999.

CHAPTER VI

COMMUNICATING AT THE END OF LIFE

Mary Ersek, PhD, RN
Marty Richards, MSW, LICSW

Adapted from: Ersek M, Richards M. Communicating at the End of Life.
In: Ersek M, ed. *Core Curriculum for the Hospice and Palliative Nursing Assistant,*
Dubuque, IA: Kendall Hunt, 2003:59–69.

I.   Basic Concepts of Communication

A.   Defining Communication

1.   Communication: exchange of information in which meaning is shared

2.   Communication has two parts: sending and receiving

3.   Communication is both verbal and nonverbal

B.   Verbal Communication

1.   What someone says

2.   Also includes other verbalizations, for example, moans, groans, sighs

3.   When people have lost their ability to speak because of aphasia or other problems, their ability to understand and respond in ways other than verbal often remains good; don't assume a lack of understanding

C.   Nonverbal Communication

1.   Nonverbal communication includes

    a)   How a person sits or stands

    b)   Gestures

    c)   How a person moves

    d)   Facial expressions

        e)   Tone of voice

        f)   Appearance such as clothing, hair, jewelry, etc.

        g)   Eye contact (or lack of eye contact)

        h)   Touching the person (or lack of touching)

2.   Touch

        a)   Important nonverbal communication skill

        b)   For some people, gentle touch can communicate support, respect, care

        c)   For others, touching invades personal space and is threatening

        d)   Let the other person take the lead; watch the person's response to initial touch to decide whether to use this communication approach

3.   The role of silence in communication[1]

        a)   Doesn't always mean the person doesn't want to talk; may mean that they are in deep thought about something painful or sensitive; give the person time without making him or her feel rushed

        b)   Sometimes you may not know what to say; at other times, there isn't anything to say; in these situations, saying nothing and remaining close can offer more comfort than words; this is called "presence" or "being present"

        c)   Learn to be comfortable with silence especially when working with patients and families at the end of life (EOL)

D. Basic Communication Skills: Setting the Environment

1.   Ensure that the person can see you, especially your face

2.   Get at eye level with the person

3.   Go to or create a quiet, private place; ask to turn off the radio or TV; close door if possible

4.   Take into account vision and hearing problems that may hinder communication

E. Basic Communication Skills: Listening[2-3]

1.   Active process of receiving, paying attention to, and making meaning of what another person is communicating

2.   To listen, you must stop talking

3.   Guide for listening

        a)   Face the person and maintain eye contact, if culturally appropriate

        b)   Make sure your nonverbal communication "says" to the person "I am listening": lean toward the person, nod your head, murmur "mmm," don't cross your arms

        c)   Acknowledge what the person is telling you by making comments such as, "I see," or, "tell me more"

        d)   Make sure you understand what you are hearing; ask the person to clarify what he or she is saying, but don't interrupt; ask, "So you mean that..." or, "If I understand what you're saying, you're feeling..."

F.   Basic Communication Skills: Speaking

    1.   Be sure that the person you are speaking with understands who you are and your role

    2.   Speak clearly and slowly, but don't talk "down" to the person

    3.   Use clear words and simple sentences

    4.   Avoid distracting behaviors (for example, pacing while you talk or listen, frowning)

    5.   If necessary, repeat ideas

G.   Cultural Differences in Communication (also see Chapter VII)

    1.   Different cultures may have different rules about communication; for example, culture influences whether to make eye contact

    2.   Culture can influence communication style; for example, some cultures tend to favor direct, to-the-point communication, while other cultures favor indirect communication, that is, they may talk in general about being sick instead of directly stating that the person has cancer

    3.   Some cultures use more expressive communication styles, that is, facial expressions and gestures are frequently used; other cultures are less expressive

    4.   Words may have several different meanings

        a)   Words that have one meaning for a particular group may have a different meaning in another culture; for example, for middle-class, European-Americans "illness" may refer to a state of poor health brought about by a disease or stress; to someone from a traditional culture, illness may be a state of poor health caused by a curse

        b   There may be no direct translation of some words into English or another language

        c)   Do not make assumptions about what a person means; ask the person what he or she means by certain words, such as "illness," "family," "faith" or "care"

    5.   There may also be different expectations about with whom to communicate; for example, there may be a specific decision-maker in the family, such as the oldest son

    6.   Culture also influences whether one talks about death directly

        a)   Some cultures believe that even talking about death can hasten that death

        b)   Can be a problem when people are asked to decide about treatments or care, such as hospice services; this belief is also a major issue in discussing advance directives, such as living wills and durable power of attorney for healthcare

    7.   Knowing what is important can be gained by using a cultural guide to determine what is expected

        a)   There is no "cookbook" about how to talk to everyone in a culture

        b)   Try to find out all you can about a cultural group, but remember that each person is an individual

        c)   Ask the patient or family what their traditions are

    8.   Work with a medical interpreter if English is not the family's or patient's first language

H.   Gender Differences in Communication

1.   Men and women may have very different styles in how they share information and feelings

2.   Culture and religion may affect social status of men and women, which in turn influences how they expect others to communicate with them

3.   Older women may defer to a husband or son in making decisions or talking about concern

I.   Age

1.   When communicating with children, consider their stage of development; in other words, can they understand abstract words like "terminal;" even if they understand the word, do they have the emotional maturity to deal with what it means?

2   In many cultures, older adults are treated with great respect; communication must reflect this respect

3.   Ask the older adult how she or he prefers to be addressed, for example, would they like to be called "Mrs. Hernandez" or "Maria"?

4.   Advanced age increases the chances that sensory losses (for example, hearing or eyesight) may influence communication

J.   Being Aware of One's Own Communication Style

1.   Know your own personal communication style so you can understand where your style may create difficulties for others

2.   Avoid labeling others because their communication style differs from yours, e.g., labeling a quiet person as withdrawn; labeling an assertive person as pushy or threatening

II.   Elements of Therapeutic Communication: Special Issues in Working with the Dying

A.   Effective Communication Is an Essential Skill for Working with Those at EOL

B.   Difficulties in Communicating with Dying Patients[2]

1.   Cultural and societal issues

a)   Denial of death; although our society is becoming more open, there still is a reluctance to speak openly about death, particularly to the dying person

b)   Having little or no experience with death; many Americans have never witnessed a death or spent time with a dying person

2.   Patients' and families' fears and emotions (see following section)

3.   Concerns of the care provider

a)   Not knowing what to say

b)   Fear of not knowing "the answer"

c)   Making a mistake and upsetting the patient or family

       d)   Fear of showing emotions

       e)   Feeling uncomfortable about being around people who are upset, sad or angry

       f)   Care provider's personal fear of dying

4.   Conditions that make communication difficult, such as stroke, dementia, hearing and vision problems or sleepiness and confusion resulting from disease and medications

C. Common Patient and Family Fears and Emotions at EOL that Affect Communication[4]

1.   Fear

       a)   Of having pain and other distressing symptoms

       b)   Of dying alone

       c)   That caregivers will not give good care

       d)   Of losing one's mind, losing control

       e)   About the dying process, death, afterlife

       f)   About losing relationships

       g)   About losing one's identity as a mother, daughter, employee, etc.

       h)   About money, loss of income

       i)   About being a burden (physically, emotionally, and financially)

2.   Anger

       a)   At the effects (physical, emotional, and social) of the illness on the person

       b)   At others in the family and network of friends who don't understand

       c)   At the financial losses

       d)   At the loss of plans and dreams

       e)   At the fact that their loved one is leaving them

       f)   That the person at EOL chooses to confide in someone other than them

3.   Guilt

       a)   At what they should have done

       b)   At what they did in the past

       c)   For needing time away from their loved one or for not being with their loved one more

       d)   At losing their temper

       e)   For unresolved relationships

       f)   About turning over the care of their loved one to a non-family member

4. Sadness

    a)   This emotion underlies everything and can be overwhelming

    b)   Sadness occurs often and can get worse with each new loss

5. Confusion, feeling that there are so many changes and they can't keep up; the patient's condition is changing and the prognosis is uncertain

6. Hopelessness and helplessness: feeling that there is nothing that can be done about a situation or that one has no control over a situation; anger can be the outward response to feelings of helplessness and hopelessness

7. Inability to accept that loved one is dying; sometimes family members refuse to discuss dying or hospice care with the dying patient

8. Laughter, love, and joy

    a)   These can still be shared

    b)   Humor is a gift to one's sanity

    c)   Often sharing something "spiritual" is a way to connect

D. Therapeutic Communication with Dying Patients and Their Families: Basic Concepts

1. Being present is more important than "Saying the right thing" often there is nothing to say

2. Encourage reminiscing[1]

    a)   Give patients and families an opportunity to reminisce and tell their stories

    b)   Provides reassurance that their lives have meaning

    c)   Helps to take the focus off the difficulties that patients and families are presently facing

    d)   Be ready and willing to listen to the sadness that may come with reminiscing

3. Care providers don't have all the answers; it's okay to say "I don't know."

4. Important messages to communicate: (adapted from[1])

    a)   "I will listen to you."

    b)   "I will be honest and truthful with you."

    c)   "I will not abandon you."

    d)   "I value you as a person."

    e)   "I will respect your values and goals and help you to achieve those goals as much as I am able."

    f)   "I will give you every chance to ask questions. If I don't know the answer to your question, I'll try to find someone who does have the answer."

    g)   "I accept that you will at times be sad, frightened, or angry. I will not turn away or avoid you when you are experiencing these emotions."

    h)   "When caring for you or your loved one, I will ask myself, 'What would I do if this were my family member?'"

5.   Other messages that caregivers and family should try to communicate to people before they die[4]

    a)   I love you

    b)   Thank you

    c)   I forgive you

    d)   Please forgive me

    e)   Goodbye

6.   Make sure there is a good match between verbal and nonverbal messages; for example, telling the patient that they can trust you, but often failing to answer their call light is *not* a good match between words and actions

E.   Timing

1.   Make sure that someone is physically comfortable as you begin to talk with him or her

2.   Be aware of the times that patients want to talk about certain things; respect their wishes when they don't want to talk; use their timetables, not your own

3.   Watch medication times for the most pain-free opportunities to talk

4.   Watch for teachable moments when families and patients are most open to talking

F.   Asking Questions

1.   Remember that people have limited energy for things that have little importance to them

2.   Limit questions by focusing on the patient's or family's concerns; don't ask questions if you really don't need or want to know the answer

3.   Questions should show that you are really interested in the patient's situation

4.   Remember to respect the privacy of their feelings, one of the few things they have left

5.   If you need to ask a sensitive question, explain why you are asking the question

G.   Fostering Hope without Making False Assurances[5]

1.   Many providers wonder how they can help patients and families maintain hope at EOL

2.   The EOL can seem like a hopeless time because the hope for a cure is destroyed; however, research shows that hope often is maintained and can increase at EOL[6-8]

3.   How providers interact with patients and families can increase or decrease their hope

4.   Hope can be thought of as having four dimensions[9]

    a)   **Experiential:** dimension in which people accept and move beyond their current suffering to find joy and meaning

    b)   **Rational thought:** thinking, planning process in which people make goals and take steps to meet those goals; goals can be short term (for example, to have pain managed during family visits) or long term (for example, to live until a grandson's graduation); goals change as disease progresses

c) **Relational:** connectedness with others; people can become more or less hopeful, depending on their relationships; for example, being cut off from close family members can decrease hope

d) **Spiritual:** Involves people looking outside of themselves at the greater whole, something "bigger" than themselves; spirituality may involve religious beliefs focused on a deity, and also includes people's connection to nature or the universe

5. Ways to support patients' and families' hope at EOL[3,5]

a) **Experiential:** prevent and treat EOL symptoms; use humor as appropriate; support patient and family in using positive self-talk (e.g., "We are strong," "We can handle this," "We are together in this"); encourage reminiscing; help engagement in meaningful aesthetic activities such as playing or listening to music or doing art

b) **Rational thinking:** assist patient and family to identify, obtain and revise specific goals; help in identifying resources to meet goals; help patient and family maintain a sense of control; provide accurate information about the patient's condition; help patient and family identify past successes

c) **Relational:** provide time for patient's relationships; affirm patient and family's self-worth; establish and maintain an open, respectful connection; assure the patient and family that you accept them and will not abandon them

d) **Spiritual:** help patient and family participate in religious rituals; facilitate visits with clergy

H. Patients' Communication at EOL[10]

1. Often, dying patients and their families need to share memories and emotions

2. Sometimes people use symbols to express their feelings or their understandings about their own living and dying; for example

a) Patient talks about meeting and talking with others who have died before them

b) Patient insists that the dead person is "waiting for me"

c) Patient talks about needing to get "a ticket for the train"

d) Messages may indicate that the person knows that death is near and that he or she is ready to die

3. Some patients may need to talk with others to settle relationships and say they're sorry for past actions

I. Educating and Supporting Families and Patients in Terminal Illness

1. Help people understand the importance of sharing with each other at EOL

2 Education can take place formally and informally

3. Educate and support patients and families by role modeling effective communication skills

4. Use written materials so the patient and family have a resource to review

III. Dealing with Conflict[3]

A. **The crisis of a terminal illness can bring issues to the surface and result in open family conflicts; you may get caught right in the middle of it; remember that in these situations**

1. There are many sides to every situation

2. Do not take sides

3. Remember that you see only a snapshot in the whole moving picture of the family's interactions

4. Sometimes, conflict is expressed to or directed at other family members because these people are "safe" and patients know that they will be forgiven as part of unconditional love that exists in some families

5. Grief can be expressed as anger

6. Sometimes, anger is directed at healthcare team members

B. **Dealing with patient or family anger directed at healthcare provider**

1. Tips for managing your own responses[3]

   a) Take an emotional step back from the situation; if you can, physically get away from the situation

   b) Think about your emotions: what exactly are you feeling? Anger? Fear? Sadness? Something else?

   c) Do any of the emotions you're feeling show themselves in your actions? How?

   d) Talk with other team members about how you are feeling; together, try to figure out what the conflict is about and who is involved

   e) Talk with the other people involved in the conflict; make a plan for dealing with the conflict or disagreement

   f) Always use "I" statements (e.g., "I am trying to understand what you would like me to do," or "I feel uncomfortable when you raise your voice")

2. When you communicate with someone who is angry or distressed, remember the following[2]

   a) Recognize frustrating and frightening situations; put yourself in the person's situation. How would you feel? How would you want to be treated?

   b) Treat the person with respect

   c) Answer the person's questions clearly; if you cannot answer the questions, consult with other team members

   d) Keep the person informed; tell the person what you are going to do and why

   e) Do not keep the person waiting for long periods; address the person's questions and concerns as quickly as possible

   f) Stay calm

g) Recognize that families and patients need to express their grief and frustration; remember that anger is a normal part of the grieving process

h) Do not argue with or touch the person

i) Use active listening skills; let the person express any angry feelings

j) Protect yourself from violent behaviors by standing at a safe distance, etc.

k) Report the person's behavior to other team members

CITED REFERENCES

1. American Association of Colleges of Nursing and the City of Hope National Medical Center. Module 6: Communication. End-of-Life Nursing Education Consortium (ELNEC) project; 2003. Funded through the Robert Wood Johnson Foundation.

2. Sorrentino S, Gorek B. *Mosby's Textbook for Long-Term Care Assistants,* 4th ed. St. Louis: Mosby; 2003:76, 88–95.

3. Richards M, Ersek M. *Communication at the End-Of-Life. Palliative Care Resource Education Team (PERT) Train-The-Trainer Curriculum.* Seattle (WA): Swedish Medical Center; 2004.

4. Byock I. Dying well: *The Prospects for Growth at the End of Life.* New York: Riverhead Books; 1997.

5. Ersek M. The meaning of hope in the dying. In: Ferrell BR, Coyle N, eds. *Textbook of Palliative Nursing.* 2nd ed. New York: Oxford University Press; in press.

6. Herth K. Fostering hope in terminally-ill people. *J Adv Nurs* 1990;15:1250–1259.

7. Herth K. Hope in the family caregiver of terminally-ill people. *J Adv Nurs* 1993;18: 538–548.

8. Ritchie MA. Self-esteem and hopefulness in adolescents with cancer. *J Pediatr Nurs* 2001;16:35–42.

9. Farran CJ, Herth KA, Popovich JM. *Hope and Hopelessness: Critical Clinical Concepts.* Thousand Oaks, CA: Sage; 1995.

10. Callanan M, Kelley P. *Final Gifts: Understanding the Special Awareness, Needs, & Communications of the Dying.* New York: Bantam Books; 1997.

ADDITIONAL REFERENCES AND RESOURCES

Palliative Care Resource Team (P.E.R.T.) [website]. Accessed June 1, 2004. Available from: URL: http://www.swedishmedical.org/PERT.htm.

Rosenblum D. Listening to people with cancer. *Sem Oncol.* 1994;Dec;21:701–4.

Zen Hospice Project [website]. Accessed June 1, 2004. Available from: URL: http://www.zenhospice.org.

CHAPTER VII

CULTURAL CONSIDERATIONS IN END-OF-LIFE CARE

Sarah A. Wilson, PhD, RN

Adapted from: Wilson SA. Cultural Considerations at the End of Life.
In: Ersek M, ed. *Core Curriculum for the Hospice and Palliative Nursing Assistant,*
Dubuque, IA: Kendall Hunt, 2003:71–84.

I.   Culture

A.   Definitions

1.   There are many different definitions of culture. Culture was first defined in 1871 by Edward Tylor, a British anthropologist, as the complex whole, which includes knowledge, beliefs, art, morals, law, custom, and any other capabilities, and habits acquired by a person as a member of society[1]

2.   Madeline Leininger, a nurse anthropologist, defined culture as the values, beliefs, norms, and practices of a particular group that are learned and shared and guides our thinking, decisions, and actions in a patterned way[2]

3.   Culture is a way of perceiving, behaving, and evaluating the environment and provides a blueprint for determining values, beliefs, and practices[3]

4.   Culture guides our thinking, doing, and being and is shared by members of the same cultural group[4]

B.   Characteristics of Culture[3-5]

1.   Culture functions as a whole, a change in one part affects the other parts

2.   Culture is socially learned and shared by members of a group; certain values and ideas are shared. Culture is not transmitted genetically

3.   Culture is dynamic and constantly changing. Culture enables humans to adapt to changes in the environment, resources, and technology

4.   Culture is universal; all humans have culture

5. Culture often exists at an unconscious level or implicit level

6. People may belong to more than one cultural group. Culture may include a religious group, a professional group, age group, or an ethnic group. For example, someone may be a member of the Roman Catholic culture, the culture of vocational nurse, a baby-boomer or a member of the Asian culture

C. **Concepts and Terminology Related to Culture[4-6]**

1. Ethnicity or ethnic group[4]

   a) Refers to groups whose members share a common social and cultural heritage that is passed down to each generation

   b) Members of an ethic group have a sense of "shared people hood," or a sense of a common identity

2. Acculturation

   a) The process of adapting to another culture, modifying or changing one's culture as a result of contact with another culture. Example, changing language to speak English

   b) Factors that may influence acculturation are age, education, length of time in this country, income or socioeconomic status, and religion

3. Diversity

   a) Refers to difference in race, ethnicity, national origin, age, religion, gender, sexual orientation, social and economic class or status, education and related attributes of groups of people[5]

4. Race[4-6]

   a) Concept that refers to physical and biological differences. Members of a group that share certain physical traits such as skin color, bone structure, or blood

   b) Concept of biological race is not consistent with scientific data and does not explain human variation

   c) All humans are very similar, 99.9% at the DNA level

   d) Race has been used to classify people into groups and treat certain groups unfairly

   e) United States Census 2000 for the first time gave respondents the option of selecting one of more race category to indicate their racial identities.[7] Race and Hispanic origin are considered as two separate categories by the 2000 census. Hispanic may be of any race

5. Racism is belief that members of one race are superior to another race

6. Prejudice is an unjustified negative attitude based on a person's group membership

7. Stereotype is the belief that all people from a given group are the same and share the same values and beliefs or characteristics

8. Ethnocentrism is the tendency of people to believe their ways of thinking, acting, and believing are the only right and proper ways[5]

D.   Why is culture important to study?

1.   Changing population demographics in the United States

    a)   White majority population is aging and shrinking. The Black, Hispanic, Asian and American Indian populations are young and growing[4]

    b)   US is a multicultural society made up of many different ethnic groups. According to the 2000 census[7] the US population distribution is

        i.   White 77.3%

        ii.   Black or African American 11.9%

        iii.   American Indian & Alaska Native 0.8%

        iv.   Asian 3.8%

        v.   Hispanic or Latino of any race 12.6%

    c)   Spanish/Hispanic/Latino population has increased 57.9% in the past decade[7]

    d)   Immigration patterns into US have changed. Prior to the 1940s most immigrants were from Europe. New immigrants are from Mexico, Philippines, China, India, Brazil, Pakistan, Japan, Turkey, Egypt, and Thailand[4]

2.   Cultural identity is integral to all aspects of life

3.   Culture influences how people define health and illness, who they consult for health problems, how they care for the sick, and the practices used to stay healthy

4.   Beliefs about death and dying are an integral part of culture

5.   Helps us to plan and deliver care that is culturally sensitive and appropriate

6.   Helps us to learn about our own culture and how it influences our behavior

II.   Cultural Sensitivity and Cultural Competence[8-10]

A.   Cultural sensitivity and cultural competence are different

1.   Cultural sensitivity is an awareness of differences among groups. Relates to personal attitudes such as not saying things that are offensive

2.   Cultural competence is the incorporation of one's cultural diversity experience, awareness, and sensitivity into everyday practice behaviors.[9] It goes beyond cultural awareness or sensitivity. Culture competence combines knowledge, attitudes, acquired skills, and behavior.[10] It is an approach

    a)   Culturally competent healthcare providers

        i.   Are willing to learn and ask questions

        ii.   Keep an open mind, avoid making assumptions and judgments

        iii.   Learn from mistakes

        iv.   Appreciate differences in people

        v.   Recognize building relationships takes time

        vi.   Have a desire to be culturally competent

B. **Culturally competent healthcare is based on the uniqueness of a person's culture; includes cultural norms and values**

C. **Barriers to cultural competence**

 1. Biases, known & unconscious

 2. Lack of knowledge of other cultures

 3. Lack of desire to become culturally competent

 4. Lack of exposure to other cultures

III. **Cultural Values in the United States**

A. **Dominant Values**

 1. Achievement & success

 2. Competition

 3. Freedom

 4. Individualism and individuals making decisions

 5. Work

 6. Progress

 7. Youth and beauty

 8. Volunteerism, helping others in times of need

B. **Values of US Healthcare System**

 1. Scientific medicine, based on scientific facts

 2. Use of technology to treat disease or stop progression of disease

 3. Cure, the ability to eliminate or correct the problem

 4. Autonomy and truth telling, informing the patient of the nature of the illness and the likelihood of recovery

IV. **Models for Cultural Assessment[3-5]**

A. **A cultural assessment may be defined as a systematic appraisal of individuals, groups, and communities**

B. **A number of different models exist for a cultural assessment**

C. **Most models include information about communication, nutrition, education, family patterns, religious preference, ethnic affiliation, time perceptions, space and biological variations**

D. Fong's[3] CONFHER model is practical and easy to use. CONFHER includes

1. C = Communication

   a) Does the patient read and speak English? Does the patient understand common health terms such as "pain" or "fever"?

   b) Is an interpreter needed?

   c) Nonverbal behavior such as facial expression, eye contact when speaking, body language, and comfortable space between individuals when talking

   d) Examples of communication: Native Americans avoid eye contact and value silence. Japanese Americans bow head when greeting to show respect and speak softly. African Americans are very expressive in communication

2. O = Orientation

   a) What is the person's ethnic identity, value orientation and acculturation?

   b) What group does the person identify with? For example, Asian, Chinese, African American?

   c) Where were they born?

   d) What is their value orientation?

      i. Relationship of humans and nature

      ii. Purpose in life

      iii. Time orientation. Past, present or future oriented?

   e) Examples of orientation. American Indians value the past and believe humans should live in harmony with nature

3. N = Nutrition

   a) Food preferences and taboos

   b) Meaning of food, association with certain events or celebrations. For example, people may have special food for Christmas, Chanukah, or birthdays

   c) Food is source of comfort and love

   d) Ask people if there are any foods that they must avoid. For example, eating pork is a taboo for Jewish or Muslims persons

4. F = Family relationships

   a) Family structure. Who is in the family? What are family member's roles? Roles of children, older adults, gender differences in roles. Who is the head of the household? Who takes care of children?

   b) Family dynamics. How does the family function and complete tasks. How are decisions made? Who manages finances? Is it important to have family present when someone is sick?

   c) What goals are important to family?

   d) Example. Asian families value and respect elders, children are expected to be loyal to the family and care for family members. African Americans have a strong family orientation, it is important for family to be present when someone is sick

5.   H = Health and health beliefs

   a)   Health beliefs refer to convictions that influence health behavior. What the person believes about health and the cause of health problems or disease

   b)   Questions related to health beliefs include

      i.   What does the person do to stay healthy?

      ii.   Who would they consult if they have a health problem?

      iii.   How does the person explain illness? What causes illness? Some explanations include, a virus, something being out of balance, evil spirits, or a punishment from God

      iv.   How does the person respond to health problems? Is the person stoic and tries not to show emotion? Or is the person expressive and openly displays emotions? For example, how does the person respond to pain? Does the person want analgesics? Do they believe that pain should be endured?

      v.   Examples of health and illness beliefs: Chinese American may believe that health and a happy life can be maintained if there is a balance between yin and yang. Heaven is yang; the earth is yin. The concept of qi, a vital force of life, is central to traditional Chinese medicine. The focus of health is having a healthy body, a healthy mind and a healthy spirit. Chinese may use herbal therapy or acupuncture along with Western medicine. Many Chinese fear death and avoid talking about it

6.   E = Education

   a)   Education refers to a person's cognitive style and completion of a program of learning. Considerations include

      i.   How does the person learn best? Visual aids? Printed materials? By watching and doing?

      ii.   How much formal education did the person complete? High school? Technical school? College? Degrees earned?

      iii.   Occupation or profession

   b)   Examples: an older adult may learn best by doing, have less than a high school education, and be a successful owner of a business. A younger adult may learn best by audio-visual aids, have a college education, a bachelor's degree and be employed as a physical therapist

7.   R = Religion

   a)   Religious beliefs and practices

   b)   Question to consider

      i.   Does the person believe in God or gods?

      ii.   What is the person's religious preference?

      iii.   Does the person have any beliefs or practices that may have an impact on health and healthcare?

      c)   Examples: Jehovah's Witness do not believe in blood transfusions. A Roman Catholic patient may want to have the Sacrament of the Sick. A Christian Scientist believes in spiritual healing and does not believe in using medications

V.   Culture and End of Life[11-13]

  A.   Dying and death are universal life experiences. Death is something we all experience, yet we know very little about it

  B.   Death systems of some type are found in every society.[5,11,12,13] **Death system is defined as "the interpersonal, sociocultural, and symbolic network through which an individual's relationship to mortality is mediated by his or her society"**[13]

  C.   Death system is made up of people, times, places, objects and symbols. The death system in our culture seems to act to keep death at a distance. We avoid talking about death and our death system supports denial of death

    1.   People—individuals have roles related to death. Examples: funeral director, life insurance agent, and florist

    2.   Time—occasions associated with death. Examples: Good Friday, Memorial Day, the anniversary of a death

    3.   Places—specific locations that have an association with death. Examples: a cemetery or funeral home

    4.   Objects—things that are linked to death. Examples: a death certificate, tombstones, death notices in newspaper

    5.   Objects or actions that signify death. Examples: a black armband, a skull and crossbones, certain organ music

  D.   Functions of a death system are to

    1.   Give us warnings and predictions of danger. Examples: sirens, flashing lights

    2.   Prevent death. Examples: police officers or emergency care personnel

    3.   Care for the dying. Example: a hospice

    4.   Dispose of the dead. Example: funeral industry

    5.   Work toward social consolidation after death. Examples: work of funeral industry and cemeteries

    6.   Make sense of death. Example: religious systems

    7.   Bring about socially sanctioned killing. Examples: capital punishment, training for war

  E.   September 11, 2001 and functions of death system[12]

    1.   Warnings not given priority, attack occurred without warning. Failed to prevent death on airplanes and ground. First responders reduced number of causalities

    2.   Caring for dying. Many causalities occurred on the scene, emergency workers provided care. Many volunteers providing aid and assistance

3.   Disposing of the dead. Very long and stressful process

4.   Social consolidation after death. Delay in stress and grief for many families because bodies not found. American people responded with compassion

5.   Making sense of death. Major issue after unexpected deaths. Personal reflection of own death. Renewed sense of national unity. Many memorial services held

6.   Killing. Shift to war on terrorism after being victims of external death system

VI.   Culture and End-of-Life Decision Making[11,13-15]

A.   **American cultural belief in self determination and autonomy includes people making their own decisions about end-of-life care**

B.   **People should be told the truth about their illness in order to make an informed decision**

C.   **The passage (1991) of the Patient Self-Determination Act was based on wide spread acceptance of belief that everyone should have an advance directive[16,17]**
   1.   No studies have shown that advance directives facilitate end-of-life decision making or guide care
   2.   The Study to Understand Prognoses and Preferences for Outcomes and Risk of Treatment[18] (SUPPORT) was a concentrated intervention study to improve shared decision making in seriously ill adults. The intervention failed to make any improvements in patient involvement in end-of-life care and decision making

D.   **Many cultural groups in the US may not share these views about autonomy and end-of-life decision making**

E.   **Older adults may believe the physician knows best and should be the decision maker**

F.   **Older adult may choose to defer to adult children to make decisions for them**

G.   **Some groups believe telling a person their prognosis is harmful because it takes away hope. Talking about death may make it happen**

H.   **Persons with a disability are fearful of advance directives because they believe they would be denied care**

I.   **Minority groups or people of color who have experienced discrimination in healthcare are fearful that signing an advance directive would mean no care**

VII. Selected Multicultural Views of End-of-Life Decision Making[4,5,12]

A. American Indians believe truth telling violates their tradition and talking about bad things makes them happen. Beliefs vary by tribal groups

B. African Americans are not likely to complete an advance directive. As a group they have experienced oppression and discrimination and would question why end of life care would be any different. The family usually makes decisions about healthcare

C. Asian Americans. The family is the primary decision maker. Families are unlikely to tell a seriously ill person they are dying. They believe protecting someone from the truth allows him or her to have hope

D. Mexican Americans have a very strong family orientation. Family members bear the responsibility of hearing bad news and protecting the family member. Spiritual orientation is important and they want the family member to receive sacraments from a priest

E. Healthcare providers need to be careful about assuming all members of a group share the same beliefs and values about advance directives. It is important to learn about the individual patient's values

VIII. Culture and End-of-Life Symptom Management[4,5,12]

A. **Responses to Pain**

1. Culture influences responses to pain and the emotions people use to express pain

2. Some cultures allow open and free expression of pain; other cultures avoid the expression of emotions and pain

3. Gender may influence expression of pain. American males are socialized not to express emotions such as crying

B. **Meaning of Pain**

1. The word pain is derived from Greek word for penalty. Helps to explain the association between pain and punishment in Judeo-Christian thought[4]

2. Pain is a part of life. Example: Navajo consider pain a way of life

3. Pain assessments should include the cultural meaning of pain

C. **Pain Management**

1. Majority of older adults in nursing homes have untreated or under treated pain. Many older adults believe pain is part of being old

2. Culture influences response to pain. For example: facial expressions, requests for relief of pain, and verbalizations about pain

3. Alternative and complementary therapies may be used to treat pain. Example: acupuncture, relaxation techniques, yoga, and meditation. Ask clients what they use to decrease pain? What has been helpful?

D.   **Nutrition**[19]

1.   Food and liquids are essential to life and are associated with nurturing and comfort

2.   Decisions about artificial nutrition and hydration are controversial. Some families believe that not providing food and fluids is inhumane and results in a painful death by starvation

3.   Cultural groups may have beliefs specific to food and hydration

4.   Artificial nutrition and hydration are not likely to promote comfort or enhance quality of life for most terminally ill patients[19]

5.   Nurses should provide families and clients with information on food and hydration so they can make an informed decision

IX.   **Cultural Responses to Death and Death Rituals**[4,5,10,12,13]

A.   **There is a serious lack of data on how ethnic minorities in the US deal with dying, death and bereavement.[12,13] The majority of studies have been done with small samples**

B.   **Need to be careful about stereotyping and assuming everyone is like the dominant culture in the US. There is more variation in groups than between groups**

C.   **Rituals associated with death are found in every society. Death rituals assist the individual and society with how to act in unfamiliar situations. They provide a meaning for a loss and function to restore social order. They provide a means for coping with loss. Funeral and memorial services contribute to making real the implications of death**

D.   **Death rituals of religious, ethnic and cultural groups are the least likely to change over time**

E.   **Examples of rituals in American society include: the death of President, police officer or member of the military is associated with a formal and elaborate funeral, burial and memorial services. The funeral services for President Reagan are examples of rituals. They included the horse without a rider and the boots facing backwards. Other examples: firing a gun, playing "taps," roadside memorials placed where someone died, members of sports teams wearing black arm bands**

F.   **Examples of cultural and religious variation in death rituals**[4,5,10,12,13]

1.   Orthodox Jews bury their deceased before sundown of the next day and have after-death rituals for several days[4]

2.   Mexican Americans hold elaborate ceremonies, (for example, a velorio to honor the dead).[4] May express intense feelings of grief

3.   In Asian American families the son may assume role of major decision maker for the family. Less likely to tell seriously ill persons they are dying

4.   African Americans have a strong religious and family orientation. It is important for family members to be present when someone is seriously ill. Openly express their emotions about the loss of a family member

5. American Indians view death as a natural process, favor having person die in a hospital so the home is not polluted by death

6. Hmong believe the person should be dressed in the finest traditional Hmong clothing so he or she will enter the next world well dressed

7. Muslims face Mecca when approaching death and recite passages from the Holy Qur'an

G. **Healthcare providers should ask families if they have any practices that are important to them when someone dies. Avoid making assumptions about what families want. It may also be helpful to ask the family who is a spokesperson for the family**

X. Cultural Responses to Death—Grief and Mourning[4,5,10,12,13]

A. **Grief is an affective response to a loss. Mourning is a culturally patterned response to loss[20]**

B. **Expressions of mourning differ among groups. Many people are reluctant to express their grief in public places such as a hospital**

C. **Grief is a universal phenomenon that is strongly influenced by culture**

D. **Bereavement is universal, however it's meaning to the individual varies cross-culturally**

E. **In American culture there is no clearly defined period of mourning. People are suppose to "get on with living"**

F. **Other cultures have clearly defined periods of mourning and follow certain rituals[4,5,10]**

1. Chinese Americans death and bereavement traditions are centered on ancestor worship. It is a form of paying respect. Belief that the spirits cannot rest until living relatives provide care for the grave and worship the memory of the deceased. The color white is associated with death and is bad luck

2. Orthodox Jews believe the dying person should not be left alone. Burial usually occurs 24 to 48 hours after death. Funeral service is directed toward honoring the departed. Shiva (Hebrew for seven) is the seven-day period that begins with burial. When mourners are "sitting Shiva" they do not work. Mirrors are covered to decrease the focus on one's appearance. The kaddish, a prayer for the dead, is said. Mourning for a parent last for one year

3. Mexican Americans are stoic and view death as a part of life. It is important for all family members to be present. Family gathers for a velorio, a festive watch over the body of the deceased person before the burial

XI. Summary

A. The United States is a culturally diverse society with people from many different cultural traditions. The population is continuing to be diverse as people are immigrating into the US from many countries

B. Culture influences what people believe about death and dying, the places of care for the sick and who is consulted about health problems. Health practices are influenced by culture

C. Healthcare providers need to be culturally competent in order to provide care that is culturally appropriate and promotes death with dignity

D. The process of becoming culturally competent begins with you having the desire to do so. Examine your biases and beliefs. Ask questions and be willing to learn

E. Avoid making assumptions. There is variation in all groups and there is more variation within groups than between groups

F. Consider the guidelines presented here. Enjoy your journey to cultural competence!

Cited References

1.   Tylor EB. *Primitive Culture* (Vols. 1 & 2) London: Murray; 1871.

2.   Leininger M. *Transcultural Nursing: Concepts, Theories and Practices.* New York, NY: John Wiley & Sons; 1978.

3.   Fong CM. Ethnicity and nursing practice. *Top Clin Nurs* 1985;7(3):1–10.

4.   Spector RE. *Cultural Diversity in Health and Illness.* 6th ed. Upper Saddle River, NJ: Pearson Prentice Hall; 2004.

5.   Purnell LD, Paulanka BJ. Transcultural diversity and health care. In: Purnell LD, Paulanka BJ, eds. *Transcultural Health Care: A Culturally Competent Approach.* 2nd ed. Philadelphia, PA: Davis; 2003:1–7.

6.   Institute of Medicine (US). Committee on communication for Behavior Change in the 21st Century: Improving the health of diverse populations. *Speaking of Health: Assessing Health Communication Strategies for Diverse Populations.* Washington, DC: National Academies Press; 2002.

7.   U.S. Department of Commerce. Bureau of the Census. ACS Change Profile for the US 2000–2002. Availiable at http://www.census.gov. Accessed June 20, 2004.

8.   Schim SM, Doorenbos AZ, Miller J, Benkert R. Development of a cultural competence assessment instrument. *Jr Nurs Measurement.* 2003;11(1):29–40.

9.   Zoorenbos AZ, Schim SM. Cultural competence in hospice. *Am J of Hosp & Palliat Care.* 2004;21(1):28–32.

10.   American Geriatrics Society, Adler R, Kame H. *Doorway Thoughts: Cross-Cultural Health Care for Older Adults.* Boston, MA: Jones & Bartlett Publishers; 2004.

11.   Braun KL, Pietsch JH, Blanchette PL. An introduction to culture and its influence on end of life decision making. In: Braun K, Pietsch JH, Blanch PL, Blanchette PL, eds, *Cultural Issues in End of Life Decision Making.* Thousand Oaks, CA: Sage; 2000:1–12.

12.   Corr CA, Nabe CM, Corr DM. Death and Dying: Live and Living. 4th ed. Belmont, CA: Thomson/Wadsworth; 2003.

13.   Kastenbaum RJ. *Death, Society and Human Experience.* 8th ed. Upper Saddle River, NJ: Pearson Education, Inc.; 2004.

14.   Ersek M, Kagawa-Singer M, Barnes D, Blackwell L, Koening BA. Multicultural considerations in the use of advance directives. *Onco Nurs Forum* 1998;25:12685–90.

15.   Drought TS, Koening BA. "Choice" in end of life decision making: research fact or fiction? *The Gerontologist.* 2002;42(Special Issue III):114–128.

16.   Teno J, Lynn J, Wenger N, Phillips RS, Murphy DP, Connors AF. Advance directives for seriously ill hospitalized patients: effectiveness with the Patient Self-Determination Act and the SUPPORT intervention. *J Am Geriatrics Society* 1997;45: 500–507.

17.   Mitty E. Ethnicity and end of life decision making, *Reflec on Nurs Scholar* 2001;27(1):28–31.

18.   SUPPORT Principal Investigators. A controlled trail to improve care for seriously ill hospitalized patients. The study to understand prognoses and preferences for outcomes and risk of treatments (SUPPORT). *J Am Med Assoc* 1995;274:1591–1598.

19.   Ersek M. Artificial nutrition and hydration: clinical issues. *J Hosp Pallia Care* 2003;5(4):221–230.

20.   Andrews MM, Boyle JS. eds. Transcultural concepts in nursing care. 4th ed. Philadelphia: Lippincott; 2003.

ADDITIONAL REFERENCES AND RESOURCES

Bhungalia S, Kemp C. (Asian) Indian health beliefs and practices related to the end of life. *Journal of Hospice and Palliative Nursing*. 2002:4(1):54–58.

Corless I, Germino, BB, Pittman, MA. *Dying, Death, And Bereavement: A Challenge for Living.* New York, NY: Springer; 2003.

Doorenbos AZ. Hospice access for Asian Indian immigrants. *Journal of Hospice and Palliative Nursing*. 2002:5(1):27–33.

Doug H, Kemp C. Culture and the end of life: Nigerians. *Journal of Hospice and Palliative Nursing*. 2002:4(2):111–115.

Kemp C, Chang BJ. Culture and the end of life: Chinese. *Journal of Hospice and Palliative Nursing*. 2002:4(3):173–178.

Nicoll LH. Sandy Chen Stokes: breaking down barriers to better end-of-life care for Chinese Americans. *Journal of Hospice and Palliative Nursing*. 2002:4(3):178–179.

CHAPTER VIII

SPIRITUAL CARE AT THE END OF LIFE

Barbara Head, RN, CHPN®, ACSW

Adapted from: Head B. Spiritual Care at the End of Life.
In: Ersek M, ed. *Core Curriculum for the Hospice and Palliative Nursing Assistant,*
Dubuque, IA: Kendall Hunt, 2003:93–99.

I.   Definitions

A.   Definitions of Spiritual or Spirituality[1-4]

1.   That part of the person, often known as the soul, which connects to a superior being, "higher power," or force such as God

2.   Awareness of a divine presence

3.   Person's sense of meaning or purpose in life

4.   "Harmonious relationships or connections with self, neighbor, nature, God, or a higher being that draws one beyond oneself"[4,p663]

5.   May include religious beliefs and practices, but does not require that one participate in organized religion

B.   Aspects of Spirituality

1.   Attributes of Spirituality[5-7]

   a)   Meaning—finding the reason for what has happened in a person's life and what is happening now

   b)   Value—what is cherished by the individual

   c)   Transcendence—moving beyond oneself and the situation

   d)   Connecting/Relatedness—connection or relationship with a higher being or faith community

  e) Becoming—reflecting on one's life that results in knowing who one is

  f) Hope—finding the good that could be

  g) Forgiveness—the need to pardon others or oneself for acts against us or others

C. Definition of Spiritual Well Being

 1. A sense of inner peace, compassion for others, reverence for life, gratitude, and appreciation of both unity and diversity[8]

D. Definitions of Religion

 1. An organized effort to express one's spirituality often through rituals and specific practices such as prayer, communion, baptism, and meditation[7]

 2. A particular way of expressing one's spirituality through certain beliefs and behaviors[9]

E. Definitions of Spiritual Care[7]

 1. Any palliative care team member's response to the patient's spiritual needs through various interventions, such as listening, accepting, talking and being with the patient and family about life and its meaning, and coordinating care with the patient's religious community

 2. Efforts to help the patient have a feeling of spiritual well-being

 3. Providing opportunities for reconciliation or relationship with a higher power (such as God), self and others[7]

II. Importance of Spiritual Care in Palliative Care

 A. Spiritual beliefs affect how a person lives and dies

 B. Spiritual beliefs affect the patient and family's acceptance of hospice/palliative care

 C. Hospice/palliative care is holistic; it deals with the physical, social, psychological, and spiritual parts of the patient and family

 D. Spirituality contributes to quality of life for the dying patient

 E. Spiritual beliefs and practices help the patient and family cope with terminal illness

III. Spiritual Needs of the Dying Patient

 A. Give and receive love

 B. Give and receive forgiveness

 C. Find meaning and purpose in one's life

   D.   Life review or telling the story of one's life

   E.   Develop hope that life can be lived fully and deeply

   F.   Develop hope for a life after death

   G.   Finish unfinished tasks

   H.   Mend broken relationships

   I.   Have positive relationships with God and others

   J.   Find meaning with one's life, illness and dying

   K.   Participate in religious beliefs and practices (prayer, Bible reading, meditation)

   L.   Accept one's self and be at peace

   M.   Die with dignity

IV. Fears or Concerns of the Dying Patient Related to Spirituality

   A.   Loss of control and dignity

   B.   Loss of personal self

   C.   Loss of family and friends

   D.   End of life as we know it

   E.   Lack of meaning in life and death

   F.   Being a burden to others

   G.   The unknown

   H.   What happens after death

   I.   Loneliness or dying alone

   J.   Pain and other symptoms

V. **Questions Patients Might Ask That Indicate a Spiritual Need or Concern**

    A.   **Where is God?**

    B.   **Why must I suffer?**

    C.   **Do you believe in God?**

    D.   **What do you think happens when we die?**

    E.   **Will you pray for me?**

    F.   **Why did I get this disease?**

    G.   **"Why" questions that do not depend upon technical answers are often spiritual in nature (Charles von Gunten)[10]**

VI. **Spiritual Signs That Death Is Coming Soon[11]**

    A.   **Lack of interest in material goods and things**

    B.   **Less interest in talking about things that are not really important**

    C.   **More silence**

    D.   **Lack of concern for appearance (how one looks)**

    E.   **Less interest in some relationships**

VII. **Common Religious/Spiritual Views on Death and Death Rituals[7,12,13]**

    A.   **The following information is general; not every member of each religion adheres to all practices and beliefs of a particular religion**

    B.   **Buddhist beliefs and practices**
        1.   Focus of most Buddhist practices is to attain a calm state of mind and to be full of compassion
        2.   State of mind at the time of death is important—patient may refuse medications that cloud the mind
        3.   Illness is a result of actions in this world or a previous life
        4.   Healing results from knowing the wisdom of Buddha

5. A temple or altar with a statue of Buddha may be in the house

6. Frequent meditation or chanting

7. Death is viewed as part of life and offers the chance to improve in the next life

8. It is important to assist the dying to let go

9. Some believe that the soul remains around the body for several days

10. Family may ask that body be untouched for as long as possible so the spirit can make a peaceful transition to the next world

C. Roman Catholic beliefs and practice

1. Central focus is to obtain eternal life with God in heaven

2. Illness may be viewed as punishment for sinful thinking or behavior

3. Use of many signs or symbols such as the cross, the crucifix, holy water, statues of saints

4. Important to attend Mass on Sunday and holy days

5. Praying is very important, may involve praying the rosary

6. The ill may receive the Sacrament of the Sick

D. Hindu beliefs and practices

1. Death is natural and unavoidable, but is not actually real

2. Death is seen as a pause in the eternal journey

3. Do not eat beef, often practice fasting

4. Physical modesty and cleanliness is very important

5. Belief in many reincarnations before obtaining union with Brahman (God)

6. Believe in four social classes (castes); person inherits his or her social class at birth

7. Body is washed, anointed, and dressed in new clothes after death

8. Body is cremated and water burial is preferred

9. Only those of the same social class can touch the body

10. Doing good deeds and giving to the needy are important

E. Jewish beliefs and practices. Content here refers to Orthodox beliefs. There are different levels of observance—Orthodox, Conservative, Reform, Reconstructionist, and Unaffiliated—that have varying beliefs and practices

1. Focus on life and preserving it

2. Death is not to be feared as it is natural and comes from God

3. Soul exists before the body and continues to live after the body is dead

4. Kosher foods are eaten and should be made available. As per the Torah, kosher refers to certain foods that can and cannot be eaten (e.g., pork is not permitted) and how foods are to be prepared (e.g., meats and dairy products must be eaten separately)[14]

5. Sabbath is celebrated on Saturday and certain activities may not be allowed

6. After death the body is not left alone until burial

7. Person's eyes should be closed immediately after death, preferably by the deceased person's children

8. Dead body receives a special washing by the Chevra Kadisha, specially trained members of the Jewish community

9. Burial within 24 hours (except no burials on the Sabbath)

10. Death is followed by seven days of intensive family mourning; this period is called Shiva

F. Muslim or Islamic beliefs and practices

1. Patient may want to use remaining time for prayer and meditation

2. Patient may want to read from their holy book, the Qu'ran

3. Members may follow strict dietary guidelines and period of fasting

4. Five periods of prayer are required daily

5. Patient will want to face east towards Mecca when praying

6. Believe that peace follows total submission to the will of God

7. Want the dying person to face death with calmness

8. Death is considered a natural process and a return to God

9. Cleanliness is important and may require bathing, cleaning at least five times per day before the required five periods of daily prayer; personal hygiene provided by persons of opposite gender may be very distressing

10. Body must be turned to face Mecca (the holy city) at the time of death

G. Protestant beliefs and practices

1. God is single being who spoke to people through the Bible

2. God protects, judges, and forgives those who ask

3. Believers have a direct and personal relationship with God

4. Focus on salvation through the gift of God's grace in Jesus' death

5. Belief in afterlife, heaven is promised based on personal salvation

VIII. Spiritual Interventions (Actions) of the Licensed Practical/Vocational Nurse

A. Reasons for the licensed practical/vocational nurse to provide spiritual care[15]

1. Spiritual needs may surface at any time and are best cared for if addressed immediately

2. Spiritual care needs do not occur separate from other care needs or only when a chaplain is present

3. Spiritual caregiving requires a trusting relationship such as often occurs between the patient and the nurse

B.   **Be a good listener**

    1.   Allow the patient and family to express their feelings

    2.   Do not rush the patient or family when they want to talk

    3.   Ask questions to encourage patient and family to talk about their beliefs, or lack of beliefs, but do not make judgments about what they say

    4.   Allow periods of silence and acceptance

C.   **Develop a trusting relationship with the patient and family**

    1.   Show an interest in patient's and family's feelings and beliefs

    2.   Be compassionate; let patient and family know you care about them

    3.   Remain present with the patient through periods of fear and suffering

D.   **Be aware of suffering and the emotional pain of the patient**

    1.   Such suffering may include regrets, guilt, failures, anger, feeling alone

    2.   Provide consistent, loving care

    3.   Report any physical or emotional pain to your other team members so the team can assist and intervene as needed

E.   **Encourage and offer hope**

    1.   Patient's goals may change but they can still have hope

    2.   Patients can hope to live for a certain event or to complete a task

    3.   Patients can hope for the type of death they want

F.   **Help the patient finish any unfinished tasks**

    1.   Talk to your team about any such tasks you identify

    2.   If team agrees, help with letter writing, making a phone call or allowing the patient to talk through a relationship that needs mending

G.   **Encourage the presence of loved ones and a minister, rabbi or other spiritual leader**

H.   **Assist the patient with life review**

    1.   Encourage the patient to talk about his/her life—special events, hobbies or interests, education, professional accomplishments, family

    2.   If patient has dementia, ask family members to share about the patient's life and what they were like before the illness

    3.   Notice and comment on photographs and mementos—ask the patient to talk about them

    I.   **Know the patient's plan of care related to spiritual issues**

        1.   If you have questions or concerns about the patient's spiritual needs or issues, talk to the team chaplain

        2.   Ask the chaplain how you can help with spiritual issues

IX. Summary

    A.   **Spiritual care is the care provider's response to the patient's need to connect with a superior force or being and give meaning to life**

    B.   **Spiritual beliefs and practices are important to hospice and palliative patients and families**

    C.   **Spiritual needs of the dying patient include love, forgiveness, finding meaning and purpose in life, life review, acceptance and peace**

    D.   **The major religions have different beliefs and practices related to death and dying**

    E.   **Spiritual care interventions of the nursing assistant include being a good listener, encouraging religious practices and life review, respecting the patient's and family's beliefs and religious practices, developing a trusting relationship, assisting with unfinished tasks and working with the team to plan and carry out spiritual care**

CITED REFERENCES

1.   Taylor EJ. Spiritual assessment. In: Ferrell BR, Coyle N, eds. *Textbook of Palliative Nursing.* New York, NY: Oxford University Press; 2001:397–406.

2.   American Association of Colleges of Nursing and the City of Hope National Medical Center. Module 1: Nursing Care at the End of Life. *End-of-Life Nursing Education Consortium (ELNEC) project;* 2003. Funded through the Robert Wood Johnson Foundation.

3.   Speck P. Spiritual Issues in Palliative care. In: Doyle D, Hanks GWC, MacDonald N, eds. *Textbook of Palliative Care.* New York, NY: Oxford University Press; 1998:805–814.

4.   Fehring RJ, Miller JF, Shaw C. Spiritual well-being, religiosity, hope, depression, and other mood states in elderly people coping with cancer. Oncol Nurs Forum. 1997;24:663–671.

5.   Stephenson PL, Draucker CB, Martsolf DS. The experiences of spirituality in the lives of hospice patients. *Journal of Hospice and Palliative Nursing.* 2003;5(1):51–58.

6.   Martsolf DS, Mickely JR. The concept of spirituality in nursing theories: differing world views and extent of focus. *J Adv Nurs.* 1998;27:294–303.

7.   Kemp C Spiritual care interventions. In: Ferrell BR, Coyne N. *Textbook of Palliative Nursing.* New York, NY: Oxford University Press; 2001:407–414.

8.   Vaughn F. *The Inward Arc: Healing and Wholeness in Psychotherapy and Spirituality.* Boston, MA: New Science Library; 1986.

9.   Altilio T, Eighmy J, Nahman E. Care of the patient and family. In: B. Volker B, Watson A, eds. *Core Curriculum for the Generalist Hospice and Palliative Care Nurse.* Dubuque, IA: Kendall/Hunt; 2002:155–180.

10. Hallenbeck JL. *Palliative Care Perspectives.* New York, NY: Oxford University Press; 2003:151.

11. Kalina K. *Midwife for Souls: Spiritual Care for the Dying.* Boston, MA: St. Paul Books and Media; 1993.

12. Kemp C. *Terminal Illness: A Guide to Nursing Care.* Philadelphia, PA: J.B. Lippincott; 1995.

13. American Association of Colleges of Nursing and the City of Hope National Medical Center. Module 4: Cultural considerations in end-of-life care. *End-of-Life Nursing Education Consortium (ELNEC) project;* 2003. Funded through the Robert Wood Johnson Foundation.

14. Kashrut: Jewish Dietary Laws Availiable at http://www.jewfaq.org/kashrut.htm. Accessed February 25, 2005.

15. Taylor EJ. Spirituality and the cancer experience. In: Carroll-Johnson RM, Gorman LM, Bush NJ, eds. *Psychosocial Nursing Care along the Cancer Continuum.* Pittsburgh, PA: Oncology Nursing Press; 1998:71–82.

ADDITIONAL REFERENCES AND RESOURCES

Bonnema M. Spirituality at the end of life. *Palliative Care Resource Team (P.E.R.T.)* [website]. Accessed August 15, 2002. Available from: URL: http://www.swedishmedical.org/PERT.htm.

Puchalski, CM. Spirituality and end-of-life care: a time for listening and caring. *Journal of Palliative Medicine* 2002;5(2):289–294.

Sherman DW. Spiritually and culturally competent palliative care. In: Matzo ML, Sherman DW, eds. *Palliative Care Nursing: Quality Care to the End of Life.* New York, NY: Springer Publishing Co; 2001:3–22.

Urbansky D, Webb G. *Cultural and Religion Data Sheets.* Louisville, KY: Alliance of Community Hospices and Palliative Care Services, Inc; 2001.

Wilkie DJ, TNEEL Investigators. Spirituality. (CD-ROM) TNEEL. Seattle, WA: University of Washington School of Nursing; 2001.

Zen Hospice Project Available at http://www.zenhospice.org.

CHAPTER IX

END-OF-LIFE CARE FOR THE CHILD AND FAMILY

Christy Torkildson, RN, PHN, MSN

Adapted from: Sumner LH. End-of-life care for the child and family.
In: Volker BG, Watson AC, eds. *Core Curriculum for the Generalist Hospice and Palliative Nurse.*
Dubuque, IA: Kendall/Hunt Publishing Company; 2002: 205–223.

I. Introduction

    A. This section is intended to assist Licensed Practical/Vocational Nurses with a practical reference and guideline for caring for infants, children and adolescents with life-limiting and progressive illnesses

    B. Guidelines are based on the age, developmental level, diagnosis and family specific needs and goals

    C. The range of illnesses, conditions and developmental levels of these children and their families cross a wide spectrum too involved for this section. A generalized approach is offered that can be applied or modified for all children and their families; however some specific information about the most common pediatric life-threatening conditions is included

II. Common Pediatric Diagnoses Seen in Palliative and Hospice Care

    A. Cancer[1]

        1. These diagnoses continue to be the second cause of death overall for children 0–14 years of age[2]

            a) Leukemia is the most common form of childhood cancer[3]

                i. 80% of all leukemia cases are acute lymphocytic leukemia (ALL), followed by acute myelogenous leukemia (AML)

ii.   Diagnosis is often difficult because symptoms are similar to those of normal childhood illnesses. Onset can be slow or rapid. Parent's often sense something is wrong however they cannot pinpoint why

iii.   The child's history may include: fever, bleeding, pain (often back, leg or joint pain), and symptoms of anemia (fatigue/weakness, irritability, pallor, dyspnea); symptoms of thrombocytopenia (petechiae, purpura, bruising easily with minimal trauma); GI symptoms (anorexia, abdominal pain, occasional weight loss, upper abdomen enlargement usually due to enlargement of the spleen and liver); symptoms of leukostasis/WBC clumping (headache, blurred vision and respiratory problems due to leukemic infiltration of CNS and lungs); infections (often lymph nodes are enlarged usually in the neck or groin area); generalized aching[4]

iv.   Management includes: following CBCs, serum electrolytes (hyperkalemia, hypocalcemia, hyperuricemia and hyperposphatemia associated with grossly elevated WBC count and/or massive organ infiltration by leukemic cells); fever, bleeding patterns, infection patterns, neurological status changes, GI changes, pulmonary changes, GU changes (painless gonadal swelling may indicate gonadal infiltrate), all pain and anxiety patterns

v.   Needs: discussion with the patient and family about the goals of treatments, desires regarding transfusions (curative vs. palliative), the risk of acute bleeds

b)   Osteosarcoma—most common bone tumor in children

i.   History may include: original painful lesion in long bone (may or may not be associated with soft tissue mass and/or local edema). Common symptoms include malaise, fatigue, fever, anorexia, weight loss, and pain. Metastasis can be indicated by respiratory symptoms/distress; pain/symptoms from other sites such as bone, pleura, kidney, brain, or pericardium

ii.   Management: follow systems noted above; follow changes in weight, changes in pain, and fevers. Multidisciplinary approach for pain and symptom management works best

c)   Rhabdomyosarcoma—most common soft tissue cancer in children

i.   History varies with anatomic location of tumor and the presence and extent of metastases: metastatic spread is via the blood and lymphatic systems, and frequent sites of spread are lung, bone, bone marrow, brain, spinal cord, lymph nodes, liver, heart, and breast; early spread within the muscle of origin and to adjacent tissue is common

ii.   If the tumor is orbital (eye) in origin history may include: orbital invasion, ptosis, exophthalmos, cranial nerve involvement (especially nerves II, III, IV, and/or VI) may be present

iii.   If origin is non-orbital parameningeal sites history may include: nasal obstruction, sinusitis, epistaxis, local pain, hypernasal speech, serous otitis media with facial palsy and conduction hearing loss. If the affected site is the ear there may be mucopurulent or sanguineous drainage; extension into the meninges is common along with symptoms of increased intracranial pressure (ICP). Seizures and/or headaches may be present with ICP

d) Wilms' tumor: is the 4th most common type of cancer in children, it is a solid tumor that develops from immature kidney cells known as nephroblastoma—a malignant embryonal neoplasm of kidney, typically diagnosed between 1–5 years

    i. History usually includes: abdominal mass, history of pain, fever, malaise, hematuria, possible hypertension; symptoms related to metastatic sites—lung, liver, brain, bone, and contralateral kidney (same kidney, opposite side)

    ii. Management: follow systems noted above; in addition, watch for symptoms related to compression of inferior vena cava; changes in fever and pain patterns

e) Neuroblastoma

    i. Origin: original mass is often found in the abdomen, adrenal gland, paraspinal ganglia, neck, paraspinal area of thorax or pelvis. Metastasis, in order of usual occurrence, include bone marrow, bone, lymph nodes, liver, intracranial lesions from direct extension of bony sites in skull, skin, and testes

    ii. History: pain, pathological fractures (high risk), abdominal masses which can include retroperitoneal lymph nodes; thoracic masses can induce superior vena cava syndrome (SVC) or Horner's Syndrome (miosis, ptosis, exophthalmos, anhidrosis); paraspinal involvement may lead to spinal cord compression

    iii. Unique issues: this is one of the very few pediatric tumors/cancers for which prognosis has not changed in the last 10 years; tumor progression and treatment often affect normal functioning

f) Brain tumors

    i. Early history (signs/symptoms) may include: irritability, lethargy, vomiting, anorexia, headache, papilledema, behavioral changes, bulging fontanels in an infant

    ii. Late signs/symptoms may include: increased intracranial pressure causing headache, vomiting, papilledema, increased irritability, decreased level of consciousness, changes in vital signs (including widening of pulse pressure, bradycardia), displacement of brain structures (herniation), seizures, personality changes, loss of sensation, disturbances in coordination, malnutrition and dehydration. Side effects of anticonvulsant therapy may lead to gum hypertrophy, bleeding, gingivitis and changes in self esteem due to change in appearance (often due to Cushing's syndrome)

2. Spectrum of cancer in children differs markedly from that in adults

a) Childhood cancer: usually involves hematopoietic system, nervous system and connective tissue

b) The following rarely occur in adults: neuroblastoma, Wilms' tumor, retinoblastoma, and hepatoma[5]

B. Non-Cancer Diagnoses

1. Congenital anomalies

   a) These anomalies account for the third highest cause of death in children ages 0–14 and create the largest group of children who could benefit from a hospice or palliative care program. They include

      i. Trisomy 13 and 18—congenital heart defects from chromosomal abnormalities[6]

      ii. Osteogenesis imperfecta Type I—genetic defect in collagen synthesis resulting in fragile tissues, fractures (may be in utero) and/or soft bones[7]

      iii. Werdnig Hoffman, Walker-Warburg Syndrome—a neuromuscular disorder that causes spinal muscular atrophy by effecting nerves in the lower brain stem and some motor neurons in the spinal cord. In severest cases, the infant is unable to swallow; most will not be able to sit up. Respiratory function will be affected. Weakness can progress slowly. Death usually occurs before the age of two depending pulmonary function[8]

      iv. Anencephaly—the soft, boney part of the skull and part of the brain are missing. The infant is stillborn or death occurs within a few days[9]

      v. Holoprosencephaly—a brain with only one lobe due to the embryonic forebrain not dividing into two separate lobes or only partial dividing of the cerebral hemisphere. Result in the severest cases is death in utero to facial abnormalities in the less severe cases[10]

      vi. Severe Hydrocephaly—a blockage of the flow of cerebral spinal fluid (CSF) results in increased volume of CSF in the brain that presses the brain tissues against the skull bone[9]

      vii. Cardiac anomalies not compatible with life or determined to be inoperable

   b) Other conditions/pathophysiology appropriate for pediatric palliative care

      i. Two major types of congenital anomalies

        (a) Malformations, arising during embryogenesis *(the development and growth of an embryo, especially the period from the second week through the eighth week following conception)* such as anencephaly

        (b) Deformations, late changes in previously normal structures due to pathologic processes or intrauterine forces (e.g., infections, hydrocephalus)

      ii. Muscular diseases include muscular dystrophy or spinal muscular atrophy; late stage cerebral palsy has significant muscular involvement usually compromising respiratory status

      iii. Children who have been profoundly injured or had a sudden acute illness event and will not have life support continued for prolonged periods should be identified for hospice consultation and support

        (a) Hypoxic Ischemic Encephalopathy (HIE) which is often due to intrauterine or birth related trauma/events are also appropriate for early referral to pediatric palliative care

iv.   Other relevant conditions include metabolic/mitochondrial disorders such as: Tay-Sachs, Menkes Syndrome

III.   Perinatal Hospice

A.   A prenatal diagnosis of a potentially lethal condition can be the catalyst for a hospice referral to support the expectant parents and other family throughout the pregnancy, labor and delivery/post partum

B.   "Traditional" hospice support and care for the baby if he/she survives the immediate time of delivery

C.   Grief support in anticipation of the possibility of death and bereavement support for the family when the baby dies and afterwards

D.   Includes the same preventative approach to minimize physical, emotional, spiritual, socioeconomic, and cultural suffering and to try to prevent the initiation of unintended, undesired, or futile interventions; emphasis is on *Quality of Life* and creating opportunities for a personalized, family centered experience, regardless of the duration of the baby's life

IV.   Differences between Pediatric and Adult Hospice Care

A.   Pediatric issues[11]

1.   Not legally able to make decisions regarding treatment; yet want to participate in decisions; assent versus consent. In many states, a person has to be at least 18 years-old to give consent

2.   The child's needs may be perceived differently by parents than by the sick child or staff thus affecting provision of care and communication

3.   May not have the verbal skills to adequately express feelings and needs

4.   Have varied conceptions of and reactions to illness and death based on the following factors: age, developmental level; family/religious/cultural norms; cognitive, intellectual and emotional maturity

5.   Has not achieved a "full and complete life"

6.   Desire a sense of "normalcy" and typically prefer to be at home versus hospital or may prefer hospital over home if this has been their primary place of residence

B.   Family Issues[5]

1.   Financial stressors: one or both parents may need to keep working, resulting in an inadequate support system. Quitting working can increase support but also increase financial stress. May be a single parent

2.   Respite often needed from being around-the-clock caregivers

3.   Parents and staff must deal with sibling's feelings, which may include: acting out, anger, regressive behavior, guilt ("I caused this"), anticipatory grief, fear, and/or problems at school

4.   Fear of being alone and/or feelings of helplessness with responsibility of caring for their dying child

5.   Adults often feel the need to protect the sick child and/or siblings by withholding information regarding diagnosis, treatment and/or prognosis

6.   Parental belief that "there must be something more that can be done"

C.   **Community/Agency Issues**[5]

1.   Must provide ongoing staff support and education regarding staff's own grief and personal issues

2.   Lack of referrals from physicians hesitant to stop "curative" treatment, who may believe they have "failed the child and family"

3.   Reimbursement for pediatric hospice care may be difficult to obtain and can be more costly than adult care, though more insurance companies are including hospice care

4.   Assessment of "hospice appropriateness" of 6 months or less may be difficult to determine

5.   Need ongoing commitment of agency to pediatric program in spite of small pediatric hospice population

D.   **Staff Issues**[5]

1.   Must be knowledgeable regarding physical assessment, pain and symptom management for infants and children and pediatric disease processes

2.   Staff may project fears for own children onto pediatric patient and family, i.e., "If it were my child..." "They should..."

3.   Must be able to recognize developmental level of child regarding cognitive understanding about death and dying

4.   Need education on the real needs of dying children, i.e., children feel pain, want honest information and worry about their condition and its effects on others; be able to focus on "the living" yet to be done within the context of the child's limitations

V.   **General Issues Related to Admission of Pediatric Patients**

A.   **Family centered approach to care**

1.   Requires an interdisciplinary, collaborative team approach that focuses first and foremost on the needs of the *whole* FAMILY as a unit, to enable them to optimally thrive and cope within the context of the child's condition as it changes over time

2.   Creates an inclusive model that optimally benefits the family and child, as the team works together to meet *the family and child's* goals for care and for *living*

3.   Typically requires a broader scope of individuals and providers, beyond the "patient/caregiver" model for adult hospice care

    a)   *Whole* family care involves support and intervention for all of the family as the needs arise. May include the child's school as indicated or that of the sibling(s)

    b)   May include Child Life Specialist, multiple medical specialists and ancillary staff such as PT, OT, play therapy, music or art therapy etc.

    c)   Bereavement care for siblings

4.   Sets a standard of involving the siblings in ongoing discussions and supports helping them understand the child's condition and clarify their perceptions of cause and expression of fears and concerns

    a)   Siblings need to be included in the circle of care and their individual emotional, developmental and basic needs met throughout the illness and into bereavement

    b)   Feeling validated and supported during the sibling's illness and offering ways for the child to participate in the experience may assist him/her in adaptation during the illness and after child's death

B.   Identify existing support systems

1.   Determine what is available and also what is needed for the ill child's and/or sibling's school community as the child enrolls in hospice/palliative care and as condition progresses, through child's death

    a)   Collaborate with the social worker to maintain contact with child's school, mechanism for classmate contact (counselor, teacher etc.)

2.   Identify all who are directly contributing to the child's plan of care; may be multiple sites or providers such as multiple healthcare providers, home care agency and case manager

3.   Identify existing spiritual and/or religious influences, beliefs and supports for the child, siblings and parent's belief system. Involve pastoral care

C.   Treatment/Intervention goals

1.   Discuss with child's primary physician and parents (and child as developmentally appropriate/physically capable)

    a)   Goals for treatment therapies

    b)   Goals that each person has, including the child to the extent possible based on developmental/cognitive level and parents wishes

    c)   Use each change in condition or new symptom as an opportunity to review child and family goals

2.   Discussion of treatment options and goals for care is essential. Discussion to clarify as much as possible, the intent, benefit, burden, and *meaning* of the treatments for all involved is critical to a comprehensive plan of care made in concert with the child, family and healthcare providers

3. Upon discussion it may become evident that the understanding and perceptions of the goals of treatments may be shared, divergent or conflicting among those involved

   a) Some interventions may be considered for continuation

   b) Others may be adjusted down in intensity

   c) Other interventions may not be consistent with mutually agreed upon goals nor do they contribute to quality of life for the child

4. When creating a plan of care with the child and family, it is very important to place emphasis on the child's (as developmentally appropriate) and parent's *desired intensity of care* and symptom management for the child

   a) This requires a thoughtful, planned discussion with consideration of timing and the readiness of the child and parents

   b) Key caregivers must participate

   c) Provide an appropriate setting for the discussion

   d) Be sure that adequate information is available

D. **Pain and symptom management: this section specifically highlights those distinctly different issues related to children and suggestions for helpful approaches**

   1. Thoroughly assess medical, psychosocial, spiritual needs and issues of the sick child, parents, siblings and even grandparents OR EXTENDED FAMILY when involved directly with the care of the child

   2. QUESTT[11]

      a) Q = Question the child. Verbal statement or description of pain is most important factor in pain assessment

      b) U = Use pain rating scales. Provides subjective quantitative measure of pain intensity

      c) E = Evaluate behavior. Common indicators of pain in children and are especially valuable in assessing pain in non-verbal children, including infants

      d) S = Secure parents involvement because they know their child best

      e) T = Take cause of pain into account because pathology or procedure may give clues to expected intensity and type of pain

      f) T = Take action to meet the established goal (child's acceptable pain level) in order to maintain acceptable pain levels through the use of analgesic/adjuvant drugs and/or non-pharmacological methods

   3. GOLDEN RULE: Whatever is painful to an adult is painful to a child or an infant!

   4. Utilize EMLA or similar product for blood draws or IV insertions to decrease fears or distress

   5. Detailed guides for pain and symptom management in hospice and palliative care are found in other chapters in this guide

   6. Safe and effective pain management is essential regardless of age and size of infant or child

   7. Fears of addiction must be addressed. Fears of using "adult" pain medications—"baby aspirin mentality"

E.   **After-hours coverage and continuity of care**

    1.   Needs of child/family should be assessed prior to admission to either hospice or palliative care program

        a)   Consider if and how the individual hospice/palliative care program can meet anticipated needs

        b)   If needs cannot safely and realistically be met with the present resources, identify additional or alternative resources in the community best equipped to handle and meet the pediatric patient/family needs

        c)   Attempt to create a collaborative framework to meet the needs of patient and family with all providers involved with child's care/family needs

    2.   For children and their families, a high priority must be placed on continuity of care

        a)   Fragmented or poorly coordinated care for the child and family can exacerbate an already strained coping pattern

            i.   The nurse can facilitate communication between the providers and the family in order to maintain the established plan of care for the child/family and to avoid frustration, confusion and duplication of efforts

            ii.   Maximizing opportunities to communicate between providers and ensure continuity between settings (home, clinic, hospital, school etc.) is an important and primary role of the nurse

        b)   As a "case manager" the nurse can keep the team and other healthcare providers updated on the evolving plan of care for the child and keep the existing support system intact for the benefit of the family

        c)   Regular reports to referral sources can maintain optimal contact with the child's care team

VI.   Developmental Considerations in Pediatric Assessment

A.   **Special considerations for examining and interpreting assessment information are necessary for clinicians dealing with infants and children[1]**

B.   **Use the appropriate pain scale for the child's developmental age. An example is the Wong-Baker Faces Pain Rating Scale (see Chapter IV)**

C.   **Appraisal of the child's developmental level is the first step toward a positive interaction, which reinforces the child's sense of security, mastery and self-esteem**

    1.   Infant (0–1 year)

        a)   Stranger anxiety is prevalent at 7 months of age and older; do physical examination with parent holding baby or within close view; smile; approach should be unhurried and gentle, use soft voice; avoid abrupt jerky movements

    b)   Pain related behaviors: increased irritability, changes in crying patterns, handling/feeding changes, usual comfort measures less effective, facial expression is vigilant or angry, withdraws affected body part

        i.   In the first few months there is no apparent "understanding" of pain but baby has response to painful stimuli. *After repeated painful experiences even the youngest infant learns to fear pain*

        ii.   Children develop anticipatory fear related to perceived painful situations, and as verbal skills develop use descriptive words for pain such as "owie, boo-boo, ouchie"

        iii.   Ask parent/child how pain/hurt is referred to: utilize the familiar words for pain in the family; plan supportive interventions with parents; child may withdraw from social or play activity if pain persists[12]

2.   Toddler (1–3 years)

    a)   Separation and stranger anxiety starts to decrease

    b)   Examine child in parent's lap, complete physical assessment through playful interactions (i.e., "Simon Says..." or puppet play) and minimize initial physical contact

    c)   Praise for cooperative behavior

    d)   Identify words used for pain and discomfort

    e)   Offer choices when appropriate

3.   Preschool Child (3–5 years)

    a)   Likes being a "helper," having choices and trying out equipment for him/herself

    b)   Examine with parent close by

    c)   Needs positive reinforcement and praise

    d)   Less tentative than toddlers although may still have some stranger anxiety

    e)   Identify words used by child to describe pain

    f)   Offer choices when appropriate and incorporate measures that the child believes will work i.e., what has been done at home, what they have seen. This can be the first step to including the child in the decision-making process

4.   School-age Child (5 years+)

    a)   Able to understand simple explanations regarding illness and body functioning

    b)   Developing understanding of "cause and effect," understands relationship between pain, other symptoms and disease process

    c)   Provide age appropriate information and teaching regarding pain regiment and rationale

    d)   Answer questions briefly and honestly

    e)   Include child in decision-making process when possible

    f)   Identify words to describe pain used by child

g)   Utilize dolls for "parallel" assessment and intervention

h)   Use appropriate picture books for aiding in explanation of bodily functions or changes

i)   Offer choices when appropriate and incorporate measures that the child believes will work

5.   Adolescent

a)   More privacy and independence needed, prefers and should be included in explanation/findings

b)   More introspective; increasing use of mental/cognitive coping strategies; has capacity for coherent understanding of physiologic processes

c)   Allow for adolescent's input, insight, choices and need for control

d)   Attention needs to be given to self-esteem and personal image as it changes over time, related to peers and develop strategies to minimize distress in this area, reinforce the positives and choices available

e)   Participation in decision-making may be influenced by culture, age and religious norms of family

VII. General Care Issues for Child/Family

A.   Symptom Management Approaches

1.   Nurse needs to be familiar with the child's developmental level to engage in any discussion on how they are physically feeling, for teaching related to care or disease progression, selection of pain assessment tools

2.   Give child and parent's choices in planning medication, treatments or procedures and their daily living regimen to fit family lifestyle and goals for comfort

3.   An important element of care for children and their families is the maintenance of NORMALCY as defined by the patient or parent in as many areas of life as possible and the incorporation of attention to physical appearance/self-esteem into daily routines

4.   CONTROL is a most important aspect of approaching care for both the child and the parents

a)   The sick child may demonstrate an increased need for structure and routine as their scope of control diminishes

b)   This is normal and should be accommodated with an ongoing attempt to give choices and respect their need for routine that reinforces a sense of safety and security

5.   Nursing visits typically involve some socialization activities with the child and siblings to create a therapeutic and relaxed environment prior to doing physical exam as a means of transitioning focus of time together

a)   Child will be more at ease when related to as a person first and as a sick child last

b)   Incorporate play into methods of communication as age appropriate

c)   Assume a relaxed posture, try to sit at child's level; avoid trying too hard which can come across as patronizing and "fake"

B.   Planning Care for the Pediatric Patient

1.   This patient population requires familiarity with and a planned response to any potential symptoms for the child's disease process and diagnosis

2.   Identify those symptoms and/or perceived "emergencies" which the child and parents fear most and have a plan in place to respond quickly to treat them across possible settings (home, hospital, school, palliative care unit, inpatient hospice)

3.   Nurses need to anticipate and prepare a plan for these occurrences to help minimize and if possible, prevent the suffering from fear of pain

4.   Examples may include

    a)   Seizure management: have necessary medications in appropriate routes on hand for children with any neurological component to their disease to respond to any possible seizure symptoms, which may cause physical or emotional distress (suggestions include: lorazepam, gabapentin, phenobarbital, phenytoin and diazepam). The LP/VN needs to consult with the registered nurse or the physician for specific medications. The LP/VN could make suggestions

    b)   Pain management is essential for **all** ages. Appropriate medication is based on type of pain, then look at appropriate routes etc.

        i.   Select appropriate routes and dosages *based on weight (mg/kg)* for infants and children

        ii.   Discuss with and provide education to parents and child on safe use, benefits of opioids for pain relief and what to expect

            (a)   Based on the medication used, assist them to create a schedule and maintain a desired level of relief

            (b)   Consider cultural and ethnic influences as well as the exposure to education in schools related to illegal drug use (DARE programs etc), which may influence perception of the use of therapeutic medications

        iii.   Consider combined strategies and/or methods for complex pain and multiple types of pain

        iv.   Assess for pain in the non-verbal child with behavioral indicators and facial expressions, appropriate pain assessment tools. Examples include[11]

            (a)   Poker chip tool (how many pieces of pain do you have?)

            (b)   Eland color tool (selection of colors to represent intensity of pain applied to outline image of child's body

            (c)   Faces scale, (series of 5 faces to represent range of pain ratings); Numeric scales (usually 1–5 or 1–10) (see Chapter IV)

    v.   Pain in children can be approached with the principles of the WHO ladder as it applies to all patients

        (a)   The **WHO's pain ladder** provides a treatment algorithm that recommends a step-wise approach to alleviating persistent pain. Each progressive step on the ladder represents medications with higher potency for increased severity of pain. The first step involves the use of mild analgesics such as acetaminophen. Each progressive step recommends the addition of a slightly stronger analgesic to the patient's current medication[13]

            1.   Step 1—non-opioid with possible use of adjuvant

            2.   Step 2—opioids for mild to moderate pain with possible use of non-opioid and/or adjuvant

            3.   Step 3—opioids for use with moderate to severe pain with possible use of non-opioid and/or adjuvant

c)   Anxiety and agitation

    i.   Minimizing stress and anxiety in the child helps to reduce the suffering and anxiety of parents as well

    ii.   Agitation may arise related to tests and procedures, strangers, previous experience, untreated/under treated pain and from fears related to his/her condition, one's future, concerns for self or family; fear of the unknown such as what will happen as they are dying, etc. and after they have died

    iii.   Pharmacologic and non-pharmacologic interventions should be used. An example of a non-pharmacologic intervention is the use of relaxation, music therapy, play therapy, imagery and visualization. Reassess pain regimen for efficacy

d)   Respiratory difficulties, dyspnea, congestion

    i.   These can be very distressful to caregivers/parents and cause restlessness in the child

    ii.   Using medication to decrease secretions may benefit the child (glycopyrrolate (Robinul®), scopolamine or atropine)

    iii.   Assess fluid intake versus output

        (a)   May need to adjust feedings if congestion continues

        (b)   Parents may need education on the symptoms of fluid overload, the inability to tolerate routine feedings in the child's current condition

        (c)   Gradually decreasing fluids based on demand and tolerance is easier for parents than an all or none approach

(d) Trial use of oxygen may be beneficial if it does not increase agitation via pediatric cannula, blow by or mask (mask is the least recommended method)

e) Elimination

i. Maintain bowel function and prevent the acute stress and distress associated with constipation and the need for invasive remedies

ii. Invasive efforts to relieve constipation are very traumatic and risky for the child especially the oncology patient with bleeding precautions

iii. PREVENTION is very important via nutrition, hydration and a preventative bowel regimen to avoid painful stooling/constipation. Hydrate as long as possible to maintain urination, avoid indwelling catheters and maintain general comfort and hygiene. Bowel regimen is initiated with use of narcotics to prevent constipation

f) Blood products/transfusions

i. Pediatric patients often benefit from continuing intermittent transfusions if they add to or maintain a desired quality of life; transfusions may help the child to accomplish specific personal goals, i.e., graduation, birthday, significant outing or other milestone

ii. These interventions may prevent a traumatic dying experience if it is expected that the child may actually hemorrhage or will die at home with that possibility

iii. The balance of benefit/burden for these therapies and the decision whether or not to provide them is a discussion to plan ahead for and review over time as the child's condition changes to review the goals of care

g) Depression

i. May not be anticipated in the dying child or adolescent, but needs to be assessed PRIOR to symptoms appearing

ii. Children show the same symptoms as adults, i.e., becoming more withdrawn, apathy for known interests, decreased tolerance to change and increased labile emotions, irritability, sleep disorders, etc.

iii. Consult with physician, social worker, psychologist or psychiatrist to determine the best approach including pharmacologic interventions

iv. Reassure parents and child that depression is treatable and not uncommon for both child and parents

v. The use of immediate onset medications may offer a more rapid therapeutic effect

C.   Preparation for the Last Days of Life

1.   Continue to use hopeful language in context of condition

   a)   Negative and consistently "death oriented" discussions are not palatable, necessary or wanted for most children and their families on a regular basis

      i.   Parents may not be prepared to make final arrangements until death is imminent or afterwards

      ii.   This may not be denial, but rather a personal decision reflecting the parents' needs and/or beliefs

   b)   Assess family's ability to handle these discussions, as trust and readiness are apparent

      i.   Forcing them may lead to conflict and hostility or even rejection of care

      ii.   Hope is always present in some form and some expression for these families

2.   As much as possible, plan where the death will take place and discuss what to expect

   a)   With the help and support of the interdisciplinary team, discuss with patient and parents where they would prefer the death to occur

   b)   Explore any fears or concerns related to the decisions for place of death and dispel if appropriate

   c)   Communicate the plan to all staff involved, especially those who cover after hours, at change of shift or assignments etc.

3.   Explore and discuss the spiritual dimension of the child's life as it relates to coping with their illness and life changes

   a)   Have similar discussions with each parent and the sibling(s) and grandparents, if available

   b)   Collaborate with chaplain/spiritual counselor to address the needs and concerns that arise during these discussions

      i.   Discuss what would bring comfort at this time and what continues to be a source of strength to each of them

      ii.   Facilitate obtaining the desired spiritual and or religious support

      iii.   Provide for rituals requested

4.   Prepare family members and child (as he/she desires) for what to expect as the dying process nears

   a)   Providing this in a written form is particularly helpful for them to refer to and to use with other relatives

   b)   Use language that is gentle, informative and based on child's level of understanding and disease process/illness

VIII. Counsel/Provide Emotional Support for Child's Grief

A. **Important to consider developmental stages as the context upon which to base explanations, education, needs assessment and relevant approaches**

1. If children have a sibling or a parent, significant grandparent etc. who is dying, the issues of their grief need to be assessed and addressed by the interdisciplinary team (IDT)

2. PRIOR to the death of a child's loved one, IDT members, including the nurse, have significant opportunities to make the child feel included, to validate concerns, anticipate grieving and address the child's desire to help and participate

3. Grieving begins upon the realization something is seriously wrong or something has changed in the family. It does not wait for the knowledge that someone might be dying

B. **Stages of Human Development—there are several theorists/theories; all believe that non-resolution of a particular stage may handicap a person in later life to some degree. Although this section is toward the end of this chapter the Stages of Human Development should be interwoven in ALL aspects of care for the child and family**

1. Eric Erikson's Stages of Human Development: all stages are considered a "crisis" that must be overcome and mastered[14]

   a) Trust versus mistrust (infancy)

   b) Autonomy versus shame and doubt (early childhood)

   c) Initiative versus guilt (preschool)

   d) Industry versus inferiority (childhood)

   e) Identity versus diffusion (adolescence); directed toward dating and social roles

   f) Intimacy versus isolation (young adulthood)

   g) Generativity versus self-absorption (adulthood); most potential to change society

   h) Integrity versus despair (maturity)

2. Piagetian Stages[15,16]

   a) Sensory-motor (birth to 3 years): infant goes through several sub stages that lead from complete self involvement to learning through trial and error to use certain acts to affect an object or a person; by age 2, toddler learns that certain actions have a specific effect on the environment; thinking is egocentric (for instance, if mother leaves, child thinks it is because of his/her action)

   b) Pre-operational (3–7 years): thought is intuitive and pre-logical (magical); thinking remains egocentric with conclusions based on what child feels or would like to believe

   c) Concrete operational thought (7–12 years): conceptual organization becomes more stable and rational; child develops a conceptual framework that is used to evaluate and understand objects in the world around him/her

   d) Formal operational thought (12–18 years): adolescent is increasingly able to deal effectively with reality, abstract thinking and future thinking; deductive reasoning develops; important ideals and attitudes develop in late adolescence

C. **Children and grief responses by age** *(note: children and adolescents do not grieve in a linear pattern but rather in a "clumping pattern" of sometimes intense periods separated by long intervals where they do not outwardly show that they are affected by the loss)*[17]

1. The infant: birth to 2 years (pre-verbal)

    a) Grief reactions: irritability, change in crying or eating patterns, bowel or bladder disturbances, emotional withdrawal and slowing of development; clinginess; do not tolerate changes in daily living routine

    b) How to help: provide secure and stable environment, lots of TLC; follow a schedule, hold and play with the child often; a consistent caregiver and maintaining routines is critical

2. The preschool child: age 3 to 5 years

    a) Grief reactions: grasp of SOME concepts related to death, time and permanence are limited and often see death as temporary; may see seemingly inappropriate questions ("Why can't we just go out and get another brother?"), indifference, physiological symptoms (sleeping, eating, stomach aches), regression, fears, imagined guilt/feelings of responsibility, wide-ranging emotions

    b) How to help: same as above; understand and accept the behavior as normal; use the correct terminology; BRIEF EXPLANATIONS; reassure the child he/she had nothing to do with CAUSING the ILLNESS or death, answer questions at their level

3. The grade school child: age 6 to 10

    a) Grief reactions: a child of this age gradually begins to understand death, but may still believe that it only happens to other people; may feel guilt (magical thinking) and blame self for death; may see on again, off again grieving, problems in school (including socially inappropriate behavior, anger towards teacher or classmates, poor grades, physical ailments), anger; at this age children are at the most risk for complicated grief—they intellectually understand death, but lack coping skills to deal with the emotions

    b) How to help: same as above; provide simple, honest, and accurate information, accept behavior as normal, contact and ask for help from school counselors and teachers, acknowledge normalcy of anger and teach ways to constructively express it, answer questions

4. The preadolescent and adolescent: age 10 to 18

    a) Grief reactions: typically, by age 12 to 14, children have a complete view of mortality; they may, however, deny that death can happen to them or one of their peers; may view death as punishment; grief at this developmental stage may interfere with the child's development of identity; may see hidden or denied emotions, so called "common and normal adolescent behaviors" may be made worse by a loss at this stage (fighting, unruliness at school, rebellion, using drugs, sexual activity, suicidal tendencies, physical illness)

    b)   How to help: same as above; acknowledge that adolescents are not adults, and do not need to act or think like adults; evaluate supports available including at school; engage school and other trusted adults for support, be aware of destructive behaviors and set limits. Continue discipline parameters to maintain appropriate behavioral limits—this actually enhances security in the adolescent. Due to the inherent ambivalence and duality of feelings, intense emotions and desires for independence and tentativeness to release feelings; peer influences; may be interested in journaling, peer groups, tape recording, artistic expression, art therapy modes of expression. Accept behaviors as grief work but address destructive behaviors

5.   Young adult: age 19 and over

    a)   Grief reactions: fully formed notion of death including how death affects him/her and changes in the family structure; may experience ambivalence and confusion about what is next for them, including the feeling of responsibility to take on some of the roles of the dead family member. Grief reactions can be manifested in physical distress

    b)   How to help: urge the young adult to focus on their needs and be able to express them to adults around them as well as peers so that others can support them; may be interested in support groups (not easy in the midst of the pain of grief!)

D.   Ten Needs of Grieving Children[18]*

1.   Adequate Information

    a)   Children need information that is clear, comprehensible and age appropriate

    b)   When they don't have sufficient information, they'll make up a story to fill in the gaps

    c)   If possible children should be informed about an impending death; they already know something is taking place

    d)   They can become anxious, maybe feel responsible or may even wonder if they can 'catch' whatever the cause of the person's death

2.   Fears and Anxieties Addressed

    a)   Children need to know they will be cared for; many children who lose one parent feel the other will die too; they fear for their own safety as well

    b)   Children who lose a sibling fear they caused the death, that they will never be able to make it up to the parents or be "enough" for the parents

    c)   Research has also shown that bereaved children who were given consistent parental guidance after a death were less anxious than those for whom discipline became lax

3.   Reassurance They Are Not to Blame

    a)   Bereaved children of all ages may wonder, "Did I cause it to happen?" they need to know they didn't cause or contribute to the death because of their anger or feelings

    b)   Younger children may experience "magical thinking" which needs to be addressed with simplicity and truth at their developmental level

---

*Adapted by San Diego Hospice

4.   Careful Listening

    a)   Children need to have a person who will hear out their fears, fantasies, and questions and not minimize their concerns

    b)   Some of their questions may be uncomfortable for adults, yet children need answers and validation. Encourage questions and ensure that the children are treated with respect. It is okay to let children know you are uncomfortable but not okay to brush off the question or their feelings

5.   Validation of Individual's Feelings

    a)   It is sometimes a temptation to tell a child how he or she should feel, but children's feelings must be acknowledged and respected as valid

    b)   Children also need to express their thoughts and feelings in their own way

    c)   Adults must remember each child's personality is unique as well as their relationship with the dying/deceased

6.   Help with Overwhelming Feelings

    a)   Children need help in dealing with emotions that are too intense to be expressed

    b)   The most common feelings expressed by bereaved children are sadness, anger, anxiety and guilt

    c)   Sometimes these feelings are acted out and adults can help kids express them in safer ways through play activities and/or writing

7.   Involvement and Inclusion

    a)   Children need to feel important and involved before the death as well as afterward

    b)   For example, it is recommended that children over age 5 be allowed to make an informed decision as to whether or not they want to attend the funeral

    c)   Children may want to have something special they have made buried with the person

    d)   Children also need to be included in rituals around anniversaries or other special times when it's appropriate to remember the deceased in a more formal way

8.   Continued Routine Activities

    a)   Children need to maintain age appropriate interest and activities

    b)   Adults sometimes need to be reminded that children cope and communicate through play activity (kids are kids first and grievers second) and its okay to do normal things like laugh, play and have fun

9.   Modeled Grief Behaviors

    a)   Learning theory tells us that modeled behavior is one of the most effective sources of learning; children learn how to mourn by observing mourning behavior in adults

    b)   Encouraging children to think about, to remember and to talk about the deceased is a rather simple but effective way that adults can influence the course of bereavement in children

    c)   Acknowledging and sharing feelings with the child in this way is very important

10. Opportunities to Remember

   a) Children need to be able to remember and to memorialize their lost loved one not only after the death but also continuously as they go through the remaining stages of life

   b) Pictures and objects belonging to the deceased can be useful reminders of who the person was and the things that were important in the relationship; shared reminiscences can also be helpful

CITED REFERENCES

1. Kassner E, Alcoser PW, Hockenberry MJ. Cancer in children. In: McCance KL, Huether SE, eds. *Pathophysiology: The Biological Basis for Disease in Adults and Children.* 4th ed. St. Louis, MO: Mosby; 2002:357–362.

2. Office of Statistics and Programming, National Center for Injury Prevention and Control, CDC. National Center for Health Statistics Vital Statistic System. 10 Leading Causes of Death, United States 2002. Available at http://webappa.cdc.gov/cgi-bin/broker.exe. Accessed February 22, 2005.

3. Kline NE. Alterations in hematological function in children. In: McCance KL, Huether SE, eds. *Pathophysiology: The Biological Basis for Disease in Adults and Children.* 4th ed. St. Louis, MO: Mosby; 2002:900–929.

4. Keene N. *Childhood Leukemia: A Guide for Families, Friends, and Caregivers.* 3rd ed. Sebastol, CA: O'Reilly & Associates, Inc; 2002.

5. Children's Hospice International, *Children's Hospice International: 2001 Informational Overview.* Alexandria, VA: Children's Hospice International; 2001.

6. Connor JA. Alterations in cardiovascular function in children. In: McCance KL, Huether SE, eds. *Pathophysiology: The Biological Basis for Disease in Adults and Children.* 4th ed. St. Louis, MO: Mosby; 2002:1048–1081.

7. Carroll KL. Alterations in musculoskeletal function in children. In: McCance KL, Huether SE, eds. *Pathophysiology: The Biological Basis for Disease in Adults and Children.* 4th ed. St. Louis, MO: Mosby; 2002:1409–1433.

8. National Organization of Rare Disorders. Werdnig Hoffman Disease. http://www.rarediseases.org/search/rdbdetail_abstract.html?disname=Werdnig%20Hoffman%20Disease. Accessed February 18, 2005.

9. Padgett K. Alterations in neurologic function in children. In: McCance KL, Huether SE, eds. *Pathophysiology: The Biological Basis for Disease in Adults and Children.* 4th ed. St. Louis, MO: Mosby; 2002:566–596.

10. National Institute of Health. NINDS Holoprosencephaly Information Page. http://www.ninds.nih.gov/disorders/holoprosencephaly/holoprosencephaly.htm. Accessed February 18, 2005.

11. Wong DL. Wong & Whaley's Clinical Manual of Pediatric Nursing. 5th ed. St. Louis, MO: Mosby; 2000.

12. Clark E. *Palliative Pain and Symptom Management for Children and Adolescents.* Alexandria, VA: Children's Hospice International and Division of Maternal and Child Health—US Department of Health and Human Services; 1985.

13. World Health Organization. WHO's Pain Ladder. Available at http://www.who.int/cancer/palliative/painladder/en/. Accessed February 22, 2005.

14. Erickson E. *Childhood and Society.* New York, NY: W.W. Norton & Co; 1963.

15. Wadsworth B. *Piaget's Theory of Cognitive Development.* New York, NY: David McKay Co; 1971.

16. Petrillo M, Sanger S. *Emotional Care of Hospitalized Children: An Environmental Approach.* 2nd ed. Philadelphia, PA: J. B. Lippincott; 1980.

17. Volker B, ed. *Hospice and Palliative Nurses Practice Review.* 3rd ed. Dubuque, IA: Kendall/Hunt Publishing; 1999.

18. Worden JW. *Children And Grief: When A Parent Dies.* New York, NY: The Guilford Press; 1996

Additional References and Resources

Armstrong-Daily A, Zarbock S, eds. *Hospice Care for Children.* 2nd ed. New York, NY: Oxford University Press; 2001.

Behrman R, Field MJ, eds. *When Children Die: Improving Palliative and End-of-life Care for Children and Their Families.* Washington, DC: Institute of Medicine of the National Academies, The National Academy Press; 2003.

Davies B. *Shadows in the Sun.* Philadelphia, PA: Brunner/Mazel; 1999.

Gellman M. *And God Cried, Too.* New York, NY: Harper Collins; 2002.

Glazer HR, Clark MD, Stein DS. The impact of hippotherapy on grieving children. *Journal of Hospice and Palliative Nursing.* 2002:6(3):171–175.

Hames CC. Helping infants and toddlers when a family member dies. *Journal of Hospice and Palliative Nursing.* 2002:5(2):103–110.

Hilden J, Tobin DR. *Shelter from the Storm: Caring for a Child with a Life-threatening Condition.* Cambridge, MA: Perseus; 2003.

Menten T. *Where is Heaven?* Philadelphia, PA: Running Press; 1995.

Wrede-Seaman L. Pediatric Pain and Symptom Management Algorithms for Palliative Care. Yakima, WA: Intellicard; 2005.

CHAPTER X

FAMILY CAREGIVERS

Tami Borneman, RN, MSN, CNS

I. **Recognizing Roles/Needs of Family Caregivers at the End of Life (EOL)**[1-6]

    A. **Terminal illness is a family experience**

    B. **Developmental stage of the family (e.g. teens, young adult singles, young parents with children, families with children in college, retired): individuals within the family unit respond differently to this experience and their relationship to the patient ultimately changes roles and functions as needed. These changes effect not only the individuals, themselves, but the family as a unit and ultimately the patient as well**

        1. May influence type of response

        2. Will effect availability, especially during the working years

        3. Concerns and problems are different at different stages

        4. May effect availability of secondary caregiving support such as extended family

        5. Effects on family relationships

    C. **Reduce physical and emotional burdens**

    D. **Provide family caregivers with knowledge and skill to enhance patient comfort which will help reduce feelings of helplessness**

    E. **Provide resources for support**

    F. **Promote healthy coping**

    G. **Help prepare for the impending death**

II. Physical Concerns of Family Caregivers[3,7-10]

A. Caregiving responsibilities concerning the patient

1. Administering medications

2. Dealing with side effects of medication

3. Providing help with or actually performing ADLs

4. Wound dressing changes

5. Managing ambulatory infusion pumps/other equipment

6. Providing presence

7. Providing symptom management (e.g., for pain, nausea, vomiting, shortness or breath, seizures, terminal agitation)

8. Notifying the nurse when needed

9. Shopping for needed items and picking up prescriptions

B. Physical concerns regarding their own person

1. Age of the family caregiver (many may be elderly)

2. Fatigue

   a) Number of hours spent on caregiving/energy level

   b) Often only one family caregiver available, no other resources

3. Sleep deprivation

   a) Caregiving is a 24 hour, 7 days per week job without any breaks

   b) Directly increases fatigue levels and impacts emotional well-being

4. Chronic illness of their own, especially the elderly caregiver

C. Interventions

1. Provide resources for help in physical care and respite

2. Use occupational therapists to teach work simplification and energy conservation skills

3. Schedule a hospice aide to help with personal hygiene

4. Assess caregiver's health status, chronic health problems and acute problems (e.g., fatigue, sleep deprivation, appetite)

III. Emotional Needs of Family Caregivers[1-3,5-6,11-12]

    A. **Help support, preserve, and/or develop emotions, thoughts and relationships with the patient and others**

    B. **Caregivers may recognize that they are in a stressful situation, they may not know how to alleviate and/or cope with the continued stress of caregiving**

    C. **Specific emotional needs/issues**

        1. Anxiety

        2. Depression

        3. Fear

        4. Lack of connectedness

        5. Lack of knowledge about the disease and how to better care for their loved one

        6. Loss of control

        7. Perceived responsibility for relieving the patient's pain and suffering

        8. Uselessness

        9. Helplessness

      10. Anger/conflict

      11. Suffering from observing the patient's disease progression and physical decline

    D. **Interventions**[1,3,7,13,14]

        1. Discuss concerns regarding future care

        2. Use psychiatric nurses and licensed clinical social workers

        3. Refer for respite care

        4. Facilitate sharing of feelings

        5. Assess for caregiver depression

        6. Help family members to *be* useful, not just to *feel* useful

        7. Help move the family's focus from cure to care

        8. Involve patient and family in care

        9. Help those involved to realize that anger is a normal response

      10. Help caregiver to fit tasks and helpers together and to be specific about what they need

IV. Roles and Relationship Needs/Issues[1-4,7,11-12,15]

A. Terminal illness impacts, to various degrees, the roles each member has performed

B. Developmental stage of each member may effect coping with role changes

C. Specific needs/issues

1. Perceived/actual lack of support from family and friends which can result in loneliness and isolation

2. Anticipatory grieving can lead to anticipatory isolation

3. Loss of sexual intimacy

   a) Physical

   b) Emotional

      i. Patient may not share feelings about this loss

      ii. Caregiver may not share emotions

      iii. Results of not sharing lead to further loneliness and isolation

4. Finances and employment

   a) Many times caregivers are having to work full or part time while also fulfilling caregiving responsibilities

   b) Expense of hiring help

   c) Financial depletion of savings/bankruptcy

   d) Some caregivers have to quit work

   e) Cost of health insurance premiums

5. Perceived inadequacies of services

   a) Can lead to feelings of abandonment

   b) Can lead to feeling unsupported not only professionally but socially as well

D. Interventions

1. Minimize isolation and loneliness through available resources/networking

2. Encourage when possible, sharing with each other or with a professional, concerns about sexual intimacy

3. Utilization of hospice volunteers

4. Meet with family members/friends to address personal concerns and to create realistic schedules for sharing caregiving duties

5. VALIDATE caregiver feelings about the burdens of caregiving and ENCOURAGE them in what they are already doing

6. Provide a resource list of support groups

V. Spiritual Concerns[2,6-7,16-21]

    A. **Differences between religiosity and spirituality**

        1. Religion is a particular system of faith and worship

        2. Spirituality encompasses transcending the material and self to a higher power

            a) Feeling of interconnectedness with a higher power

            b) Meaning through a sense of relatedness to a higher power

    B. **Holistic Care—including spirituality provides holistic care through the body, mind and spirit**

    C. **Terminal illness creates an increased sense of vulnerability and mortality for everyone involved**

    D. **Terminal illness also creates loss and suffering in various degrees**

    E. **The need to find meaning in what is happening to the patient and to the caregiver**

        1. Meaning of dying

        2. Meaning of human existence

        3. Meaning of suffering

        4. Meaning of remaining days left

    F. **Fear of the future of uncertainty and ambiguity**

        1. Life in general

        2. Own death

        3. Who will be their caregiver when the time comes

        4. Finances

        5. Love and security

        6. Loss of their role—"What will I be when I am no longer a caregiver?"

    G. **Relatedness to God or whatever represents God**

        1. The concept of "God" or a superior being

        2. Comfort can come from the fact that "God" is more than human

        3. Need for rituals, sacraments, the exercising of beliefs

H. Sense of Hope

1. Linked to a sense of purpose

2. Often directly proportional to the patient's status

3. Related to a sense of connectedness to God or others

4. Provides confidence in life after death, a sense of future

5. Essential for day to day life, especially in these circumstances

I. Interventions

1. Use active listening and presence

2. Assess past spiritual support, religious practices, and resources

3. Help construct a sense of hope

4. Pray with and/or share scripture

5. Provide, if desired, appropriate religious supports (e.g., priest, minister, rabbi)

6. Provide help on the basis of individual needs

CITED REFERENCES

1. Duhamel F, Dupuis F. Guaranteed returns: investing in conversations with families of patients with cancer. *Clin J Oncol Nurs.* 2004;8(1):68–71.

2. Farber SJ, Egnew TR, Herman-Bertsch JL, Taylor TR, Guldin GE. Issues in end-of-life care: patient, caregiver, and clinician perceptions. *J Palliat Med.* 2003;6(1):19–31.

3. Ferrell BR. The family. In: Doyle D, Hanks G, MacDonald N, eds. *Oxford Textbook of Palliative Medicine.* Oxford, UK: Oxford Medical Publication; 1998.

4. Grunfeld E, Coyle D, Whelan T, Clinch J, Reyno L, Earle CC, et al. Family caregiver burden: results of a longitudinal study of breast cancer patients and their principal caregivers. *Cmaj.* 2004;170(12):1795–1801.

5. Isaksen AS, Thuen F, Hanestad B. Patients with cancer and their close relatives: experiences with treatment, care, and support. *Cancer Nurs.* 2003;26(1):68–74.

6. Kemp C. *Terminal Illness: A Guide to Nursing Care.* Philadelphia, PA: J.B. Lippincott; 1995.

7. Borneman T. Caring for cancer patients at home: the effect on family caregivers. *Home Health Care Management & Practice.* 1998;10(4):25–33.

8. Hileman JW, Lackey NR. Self-identified needs of patients with cancer at home and their home caregivers: a descriptive study. *Oncol Nurs Forum.* 1990;17(6):907–913.

9. Steele RG, Fitch MI. Coping strategies of family caregivers of home hospice patients with cancer. *Oncol Nurs Forum.* 1996a;23(6):955–960.

10. Steele RG, Fitch MI. Needs of family caregivers of patients receiving home hospice care for cancer. *Oncol Nurs Forum.* 1996b;23(5):823–828.

11. Harding R, Higginson IJ. What is the best way to help caregivers in cancer and palliative care? A systematic literature review of interventions and their effectiveness. *Palliat Med.* 2003;17(1):63–74.

12. Vachon ML. Psychosocial needs of patients and families. *J Palliat Care.* 1998;14(3):49–56.

13. Abrahm JL. Update in palliative medicine and end-of-life care. *Annu Rev Med.* 2003:54:53–72.

14. Gorman L. The psychosocial impact of cancer on the individual, family, and society. In: Carroll-Johnson RM, Gorman L, Bush N. eds. *Psychosocial Nursing Care along the Cancer Continuum.* Pittsburgh, PA: Oncology Nursing Press, Inc.; 1998:71–82.

15. Ferszt B, Houck P. The family. In: Amenta MO, Bohnet NL. eds. *Nursing Care of the Terminally Ill.* Boston, MA: Little, Brown and Company; 1986:173–190.

16. Amenta MO. Spiritual concerns. In: Amenta MO, Bohnet NL. eds. *Nursing Care of the Terminally Ill.* Boston, MA: Little, Brown and Company; 1986:115–116.

17. Herth KA, Cutcliffe JR. The concept of hope in nursing 3: Hope and palliative care nursing. *Br J Nurs.* 2002;11(14):977–983.

18. Speck P. Spiritual issues in palliative care. In: Doyle D, Hanks G, MacDonald N, eds. *Oxford Textbook of Palliative Medicine.* Oxford, UK: Oxford Medical Publication; 1998:805–814.

19. Taylor EJ. Spirituality and the cancer experience. In: Carroll-Johnson RM, Gorman L, Bush N. eds. *Psychosocial Nursing Care along the Cancer Continuum.* Pittsburgh, PA: Oncology Nursing Press, Inc.; 1998:71–82.

20. Taylor EJ. *Spiritual Care: Nursing Theory, Research, and Practice.* Upper Saddle River, NJ: Prentice-Hall; 2002.

21. Taylor EJ. Spiritual needs of patients with cancer and family caregivers. *Cancer Nurs.* 2003;26(4):260–266.

ADDITIONAL REFERENCES AND RESOURCES

Borneman T, Stahl C, Ferrell B, Smith D. The concept of hope in family caregivers of cancer patients and home. *Journal of Hospice and Palliative Nursing.* 2002:4(1):21–33.

CHAPTER XI

BEREAVEMENT

Tami Borneman, RN, MSN, CNS

I.   Introduction: Definitions[1,2]

    A.   Grief—intense, emotional loss caused by suffering; thoughts, feelings and behaviors one experiences after a loss

    B.   Mourning—the outward signs of grief; process one goes through adapting to a loss

    C.   Bereavement—complex series of reactions following death, including grief and mourning; situation of losing to death a person a loved one

    D.   Attachment—a strong need to remain close to or, to return to, another individual

II.   Stages/Process of Grief

    A.   Bereavement is a process unique to each individual

    B.   The nature of grief[1]

        1.   Urge to cry and to search for the deceased

        2.   Avoiding or repressing crying or searching—social value of being taught to have a "stiff upper lip"

        3.   Reviewing and revising internal models

            a)   Death of a loved one can invalidate one's assumptions about the world, thought patterns, and behavior, which formerly included or depended on the deceased

            b)   The familiar world becomes rather unfamiliar

            c)   Often the process is initially resisted

C.   **Anticipatory grief**[3-6]

1.   "Process of mourning, coping, interaction, planning and psychosocial reorganization that is stimulated and begun in part in response to the awareness of the impending loss of a loved one and the recognition of associated losses in the past, present and future"[5,p35]

2.   Therapeutic aspects of anticipatory grieving involve balancing the equally conflicting emotions of simultaneously holding on, letting go and drawing closer to their dying loved one

3.   When the realization of death is reinforced by the illness progression and awareness gradually surfaces, one is said to have entered into the anticipatory phase[3]

4.   Healthcare professionals at times experience anticipatory grieving. For example, the nurse may sense death is inevitable before the physician or family. The nurse begins anticipatory grieving while others are still focused on cure or prolonging life[3]

D.   **Theoretical tasks of grief**

1.   Kübler-Ross[7]

    a)   Denial

    b)   Anger

    c)   Bargaining

    d)   Depression

    e)   Acceptance

2.   Parkes[1]

    a)   Alarm—physiological response

    b)   Searching

        i.   Involves pangs of grief stimulated by memories of the loss

        ii.   Bereaved may share having seen or heard or called out to the deceased

    c)   Mitigation

        i.   Behaviors used to lessen the pain such as talking or praying to the deceased, denying the loss, increasing activity, returning to work

        ii.   An attempt is made to make sense of the loss

    d)   Anger and guilt

        i.   Anger usually occurs during the first year

        ii.   Those with the greatest anger usually experience more isolation

        iii.   Guilt over an aspect of the relationship can be a risk for complicated grief

        iv.   Can arise from imagined omissions of duty, failure and negligence

        v.   May feel guilty of still being alive

    e)   Gaining new identity—includes recovery of lost functions, adaptation to new roles and status and completion of acute grief

3. Bowlby[8]

    a) Numbing, with possible anguish and anger

    b) Searching and longing

    c) Disorganization and despair

    d) Reorganization

4. Wordon's Tasks[2]

    a) Accept reality of the loss

    b) Experience the pain of grief

    c) Adjust to an environment without the deceased

    d) Withdraw emotional energy and reinvest in another relationship

5. Rando's Process of Bereavement[5-6]

    a) Recognize the loss and death

    b) React to, experience and express the separation and pain

    c) Reminisce

    d) Relinquish old attachments

    e) Readjust and adapt to the new role while maintaining memories and form a new identity

    f) Reinvest

E. Demographics and cultural issues[1,3]

1. Be aware of cultural differences

2. Use guidelines and manuals to read about beliefs, customs and religions

3. Elicit information from the patient and family

4. Set aside own value judgments, avoid interjecting personal preference

5. Deaths of children and multiple deaths are regarded as the most severe types of loss

6. Women generally show emotions easier than men and are more inclined to seek help

7. Age

    a) Very young—difference between permanent and temporary separations is unclear

    b) Older children—similar to adults but can be complicated by failure in communication

    c) Old age—bereavement is less often unexpected, and because of the many losses encountered, it is sometimes considered to be a normal part of aging

III. Assessment[3]

A. Integrated into the conversation with the patient and family

B. Each answer to assessment questions (not merely probing) is a potential for teaching, therapeutic response and intervention

C. Includes both verbal and nonverbal responses

D. Is coupled with nurturance, comfort, touch, gentle voice, impression one has unlimited time, and a sense of presence and compassion

IV. Interventions/Resources

A. Plan of Care[3,9-10]

1. Assessment
    a) Description of the death in the family's own words
    b) Concurrent stressors, past losses, reactions to their anniversaries
    c) Affective response (feelings, inability to concentrate)
    d) Somatic responses (sleep disturbances, poor appetite, pain, weakness, social withdrawal, hyperactivity)
    e) Support systems
    f) Financial concerns
    g) Past history of coping and psychiatric history
    h) Suicidal tendencies
    i) Alcohol or drug abuse: other substance abuse
    j) Spiritual/religious beliefs
    k) Cultural traditions
    l) Unusual experiences since death

2. Nursing Diagnoses[4]
    a) Bereavement
    b) Spiritual distress
    c) Dysfunctional grief
    d) Impaired adjustment
    e) Anxiety
    f) Ineffective individual coping

3. DSM-IV Diagnoses[12]

   a) Major depressive disorder

   b) Post-traumatic stress disorder

4. Expected Outcomes

   a) Family will begin the grief process within own cultural norms and family traditions

   b) Family will share the grief reaction and its impact

   c) Family will seek support as needed

   d) In time, family will engage in life and other relationships

5. Interventions

   a) Provide continuous supportive listening and reassurance

   b) When appropriate, elicit a life review

   c) Provide privacy

   d) Encouragement of unfinished business and assist family in achieving desired goals

   e) Encourage use of cultural practices

   f) Offer spiritual support and referrals when needed

   g) Provide verbal and written information on the grief process and what to expect

   h) Use touch, holding and presence when appropriate

   i) Be sensitive for the need for silent presence

   j) Teach relaxation techniques

   k) Use guided imagery when appropriate

   l) Provide referrals for appropriate support groups as needed

   m) Encourage social support

   n) Encourage healthy coping mechanisms (e.g., exercise and rest)

   o) Give permission to grieve

B. Complicated Grief[1-3,5-6,13-15]

1. Those at risk for complicated grief

   a) Those who have an underlying low self-esteem

   b) Having had an ambivalent relationship

   c) Having had a dependent relationship (separation anxiety)

   d) Loss of role as caregiver especially if this role brought the patient and caregiver closer together

   e) Premature death

   f) Traumatic death

   g) Sudden death

      h)   Death of an organ or bone marrow transplant recipient

      i)   Death by suicide or homicide

      j)   Death of a child

      k)   Financial loss as a result of the terminal illness

2. Examples of complicated grief

      a)   Prolonged/chronic grief—memories/conversations stir up uncontrollable weeping even years after the death

      b)   Absent grief—no show of grief and sadness

      c)   Exaggerated grief—self destructive behaviors such as suicide

      d)   Masked grief—bereaved is unaware of the behaviors that interfere with normal functioning

      e)   Depression

      f)   Post-traumatic stress disorder

3. Complicated grief can cause problems in relationships with family/friends

C. Unusual Experiences[3]

1. Bereaved having felt they have had contact with the deceased family member

      a)   Often discounted as dreams or hallucinations

      b)   Often judged as being "out there"

      c)   Actual incidence is not known, but suspected to be more frequent than is shared

      d)   Mourners may feel they are going crazy because they see or hear things others do not

      e)   May create a fear of losing reality

2. Therapeutic effects

      a)   Affirmation of the death

      b)   Completion of unfinished business

      c)   Sense that their loved one is alright

      d)   Reduction in their own suffering

3. Interventions

      a)   Encouraging sharing of unusual events, both for colleagues and family members

      b)   Do not pass judgment

      c)   Do not dismiss or label as hallucinations

V. Recognition of Staff Grief

    A. Nature of the patient/nurse relationship[3,15-16]

        1. The loss is mourned regardless of the type of relationship experienced (e.g., close, ambivalent or hostile)

        2. Nurses may become callous, but are not immune to grief

        3. Sometimes grief over a close patient relationship results in a culmination of grief experienced from many deaths

    B. Coping

        1. Good deaths

            a) Nurses cope better with what they consider to have been a good death

            b) Death considered good if

                i. Symptoms were managed

                ii. It was felt that the best possible care was given

                iii. Patient came to some resolution

                iv. Death did not violate a natural order (e.g., not a child or young adult)

        2. Deaths considered bad if

            a) Nurse/family members were not present at time of death

            b) Grief characterized as painful, complicated, distressing or difficult

        3. Anger

            a) Not an uncommon response to continual exposure to death

            b) Poorly tolerated in our culture

            c) Increased if one feels responsible for not curing, eliminating symptoms or for "causing" side effects from symptom management

            d) Acknowledging anger can help the nurse deal with feelings of depression and guilt

    C. Self-Care[3,16-17]

        1. Most important is initiating action on individual, managerial and institutional levels to help staff cope with grief

        2. Specific interventions

            a) Support groups

            b) Self-assessment of numbers of deaths and toll taken

            c) Assessment of other areas of stress

            d) Acknowledge limitations and set appropriate boundaries

            e) Don't be afraid to ask for help

       f)   Assess participation in positive aspects of one's life such as spirituality, play, sexuality, laughter, hobbies

       g)   Provide/create ceremonies and programs that serve to acknowledge grief for both professionals and families

       h)   Send bereavement cards or call the family

VI. Conclusion

A. **Bereavement does not begin after death, but rather in events leading up to the death**

B. **Nurses have wonderful opportunities to care for the bereaved through listening, assisting in communications, teaching families about the process of dying or facilitating bereavement support groups**

C. **Bereavement provides nurses with opportunities to prevent ill health and to help families find new directions for growth**

D. **Grief is changing and dynamic**

E. **Grief is experienced physiologically, psychologically, socially and spiritually**

F. **Spiritually, families have a need to be comforted by those sharing the same faith, have a need for prayer and to feel supported by God and others**

CITED REFERENCES

1. Parks C. Bereavement. In: Doyle D, Hanks G, MacDonald N. eds. *Oxford Textbook of Palliative Medicine*. 2nd ed. Oxford, UK: Oxford Medical Publication; 1998:995–1010.

2. Worden JW. Bereavement care. In Berger A, Portenoy R, Weissman D. eds. *Principles & Practice of Palliative Care & Supportive Oncology*. 2nd ed. Philadelphia: Lippincott Williams & Wilkins; 2002:813–818.

3. Brown-Saltzman K. Transforming the grief experience. In: Carroll-Johnson RM, Gorman L, Bush N. eds. *Psychosocial Nursing Care along the Cancer Continuum*. Pittsburgh, PA: Oncology Nursing Press, Inc.; 1998:197–214.

4. Duke S. An exploration of anticipatory grief: the lived experience of people during their spouses' terminal illness and in bereavement. *J Adv Nurs*. 1998;28(4):829–839.

5. Rando T. *Treatment of Complicated Mourning*. Champaign, IL: Research Press; 1993.

6. Rando T. *Clinical Dimensions of Anticipatory Mourning*. Champaign, IL: Research Press; 2000.

7. Kübler-Ross E. *On Death and Dying*. New York, NY: Macmillan; 1969.

8. Bowlby J. *Attachment and Loss*. New York: Basic Books; 1980.

9. Foley, G. *Lessons from the Bereaved: Care for the Dying*. Paper presented at the Sixth National Conference on Cancer Nursing, Seattle; 1991.

10. Forte AL, Hill M, Pazder R, Feudtner C. Bereavement care interventions: a systematic review. *BMC Palliat Care*. 2004;3(1):3.

11. Association, N. A. N. D. *Nursing Diagnoses: Definitions And Classification*. Philadelphia: North American Nursing Diagnosis Association; 2003.

12. Association, A. P. *Diagnostic and Statistical Manual of Mental Disorders*. 4th ed. Washington, DC: American Psychiatric Association; 2000.

13. Bohnet N. Bereavement care. In: Amenta M, Bohnet N. eds. *Nursing Care Of The Terminally Ill*. Boston, MA: Little, Brown and Company; 1986.

14. Kemp C. *Terminal Illness: A Guide to Nursing Care*. Philadelphia, PA: J.B. Lippincott Company; 1995.

15. Loney M. Death, dying, and grief in the face of cancer. In: Burke C. ed. *Psychosocial Dimensions of Oncology Nursing Care*. Pittsburgh, PA: Oncology Nursing Press, Inc.; 1998:152–179.

16. Vachon M. Staff stress and burnout. In: Berger A, Portenoy R, Weissman D. eds. *Principles & Practice of Palliative Care & Supportive Oncology*. 2nd ed. Philadelphia, PA: Lippincott Williams & Wilkins; 2002:831–848.

17. Lo K, Causey B, Crandall F. *Care at the Time of Death*. Paper presented at the Hospice Training Program, Largo, FL; 1996.

ADDITIONAL REFERENCES AND RESOURCES

Romesberg TL. Understanding grief: a component of neonatal palliative care. *Journal of Hospice and Palliative Nursing.* 2002:6(3):161–170.

Scannell-Desch E. Prebereavement and postbereavement struggles and triumphs of midlife widows. *Journal of Hospice and Palliative Nursing.* 2002:7(1):15–22.

CHAPTER XII

CARE AT THE TIME OF DYING

Jeanne Martinez, RN, MPH, CHPN®

Adapted from: Martinez J, Matzo ML. Care of the patient and family when death is nearing.
In: Ersek M, ed. *Core Curriculum for the Hospice and Palliative Nursing Assistant,*
Dubuque, IA: Kendall Hunt, 2003:59–69.

I. **Introduction/Overview**

   A. **Once it is determined that a patient is dying and treatment to cure the disease is no longer helpful, providing comfort care ensures a peaceful death**

   B. **Nursing can do much to make this time comfortable; there is only one chance for us to do this well for each person**

   C. **Care should be individualized to each patient's needs and goals, as much as possible**

   D. **Even very ill patients can be given control over their immediate surroundings**

   E. **Patients need ongoing monitoring of their symptoms; ask if the patient is satisfied with how well their symptoms are controlled**

   F. **Providing excellent care at the time of dying includes emotional support of family members and consists of listening and being present for people as they grieve the loss of their loved one**

   G. **The major ways to ensure good care to dying patients and to support their families is by**

      1. Making the environment as comfortable as possible

      2. Giving care with an attitude of attentiveness, compassion and concern to the individual patient and the family

3. Working with the team to avoid if possible any burdensome care, such as unnecessary weights, taking vital signs or other care that may cause discomfort to the patient

4. Respecting patient's and family's cultural, religious and other values without judging them or imposing personal beliefs

5. Working as a team member by sharing observations, reporting problems and concerns and supporting each other

H. When done well, care of the dying can be very rewarding

II. Patient and Family Needs and Goals Related to the Dying Process

A. Assist the patient to meet his or her end-of-life goals; ask patient the following questions

1. Who does the patient want to be there?

2. What are the most important needs and goals for the patient before death?

   a) Prioritize care according to the patient's (then the family's) goals

   b) If there is conflict in what patients and family members want, patient desires come first

3. Where does the patient want to die?

4. Inform other team members about the patient's and family's wishes and goals; it may take the entire team to work together to meet patient's goals, for example, to arrange discharge and hospice services if the patient wants to die at home instead of in the hospital

B. Cultural influences (see Chapter VIII)

1. Determine important beliefs and values that affect patient's goals

2. Respect the need for a patient to die on his or her own terms

3. Never force your own beliefs on a patient or family

4. Avoid judging how family members cope with loss and death

C. Family needs

1. Who is the patient's family or support system?

2. Do patient and family goals conflict?

3. Report conflicting goals and values to the team

4. Assist patients and family members to "reframe hope," for example, help family and patients to meet short-term goals focused on hopes at end of life, such as the hope to have a pain-free day, or the hope of seeing a new grandchild born

D. Re-evaluation

1. Continually reassess patient goals; help patients to decide what is most important to them

2. Continually check patients for unresolved symptoms

3. Frequently monitor the effectiveness of medications and other interventions and whether patients are satisfied with symptom management

4. Always share patient's and family's wishes, concerns and need for further intervention with the team

III. The Environment[1]

A. Immediate physical environment

1. Respect the environment as a sacred space, that is, as a place where a profound change is to occur

2. Individualize the environment; determine what is important and meaningful to the patient or family related to the following

   a) Objects and views

      i. What objects are meaningful (for example, photos, rosary beads, books, pillows)?

      ii. What should be in the patient's line of vision should he or she awaken?

      iii. What about window views?

      iv. Can the bed be repositioned to improve the patient's environment?

      v. If the patient is at home, is he or she isolated in a bedroom (and is that what they want) or is he or she in a central room of the home (and is that what they want)?

   b) Lighting

      i. Is natural light available?

      ii. Is room lighting harsh or gentle?

   c) Sound

      i. Is the room too noisy?

      ii. Does the patient respond differently to various noise levels?

      iii. Provide music, TV, other sounds that the patient likes, if that is what the patient wants

      iv. Vary the noise environment to enhance the patient's comfort and sleep cycles

      v. Provide or increase calming sounds. Decrease or stop sounds that disturb the patient

      d)   Family space in a facility

          i.   Can the environment be made less sterile or medical? Is it welcoming to families and visitors?

          ii.   Are there comfortable chairs for family members and other visitors?

          iii.   Is there a close common space for family members when they are not in the patient's room?

          iv.   Are coffee, water or other refreshments available nearby?

          v.   Is a phone available nearby, but outside of the patient's room, for family use?

          vi.   Does the environment promote privacy as much as possible?

B.   Staff behaviors and attitudes

    1.   Frequently visit the dying patient's room

    2.   Maintain a balance between giving family members privacy and being there for support

    3.   Sit down when talking with the patient or family members

    4.   Listen carefully to the patient's and family members' issues; express your compassion and concern

    5.   Stress may prevent family members from listening or remembering what you tell them; they may need the same questions answered more than once. Communicate with the healthcare team to ensure that the patient and family are given consistent answers and explanations

    6.   Recognize the importance of your presence, that is, being vs. doing; role-model this behavior for families and other staff

IV. Symptom Management Related to Decline in Status

A.   Goals of care: watch for new or note existing symptoms or problems; ask the patient which problems cause the most concern

B.   Common symptoms in patients near the time of death (also see Chapters IV and V)

    1.   Agitation/restlessness

        a)   The person may make restless and repetitive motions, such as pulling at bed linen or clothing

        b)   Observe for reversible physical causes, such as full bladder, constipation, impaction

        c)   Consider that the cause of restlessness or distress may be emotional or spiritual in nature

d) Nursing actions

   i.   Speak in a quiet, natural way

   ii. Lightly massage the patient's forehead, back, or arms, if acceptable to patient

   iii. Read to the person

   iv. Play some soothing music

   v.   Try to decrease the number of people around the person

   vi. Avoid asking a lot of questions or talking a lot

   vii. Do not interfere with or try to restrain restless motions, unless the patient is harming himself or herself

   viii. Sedative and pain medications as ordered

2. Pain

   a) Observe for moaning, restlessness, furrowing of the brow and grimacing, which may indicate pain or discomfort

   b) Continue or begin non-drug pain therapies such as

      i   Gentle massage

      ii. Repositioning the patient

      iii. Pleasant diversions, such as music, being read to, etc.

      iv. For some patients, company and distraction can help pain, but for others a calm, quiet environment works better; observe patients for what seems to provide the most comfort. Communicate this to the healthcare team

      v.   Pain medications as ordered with continued assessment for effectiveness and need to increase or decrease

3. Dyspnea

   a) Difficulty breathing, feeling short of breath

      i.   Cheyne-Stokes breathing pattern is characterized by uneven shallow breathing alternating with periods of apnea. It is a common respiratory pattern prior to death[2]

   b) Can be very distressing to patients and families

   c) Nursing actions

      i.   Positioning: put the head of the bed up; put pillows behind the patient's head; and if possible, sit the patient up in a reclining chair

      ii. Suggest that the patient move more slowly; keep still, lay quietly; and use pursed-lip or deep, slow breathing

      iii. Direct a fan to the face or open a window (or both) to move air through the patient's room

      iv. Use relaxation or distraction techniques with the patient

v.   Morphine may be ordered to help decrease the feelings of breathlessness[2]

vi.   Oxygen therapy does not usually relieve dyspnea at the end of life, though it is sometimes used if the patient and/or family think that it is helping[2]

4.   Noisy respirations or "death rattle"

a)   Caused by relaxation of throat muscles and pooling of secretions

b)   More disturbing to families than patient

c)   Nursing actions

i.   Frequently change patient's position

ii.   Provide support to the families; assure them that noisy breathing does not mean the patient is in distress; avoid using the term "death rattle" with or in the presence of the patient and/or family

iii. Medications to calm breathing or decrease secretions as ordered

5.   Anorexia and dysphagia

a)   Anorexia: lack of appetite

b)   Dysphagia: difficulty swallowing

c)   Result of the process of the body "shutting down"

d)   Can cause the family distress; conflict can occur if the goals of therapy are not clear

e)   Nursing actions

i.   Offer conscious patients small frequent sips of fluids or bits of soft food followed by mouth care

(a)   If having difficulty swallowing, a consult with a nutritionist or speech therapist may be helpful depending on condition and goals

ii.   For unconscious patients, provide frequent, gentle mouth care

iii. Help families to cope with the changes in patient status

C.   **General comfort care for patients nearing death**[3]

1.   Oral care

a)   Keep the patient's mouth moist

i.   Rinse the patient's mouth frequently with water

ii.   Keep room humidified using spray bottle or humidifier

iii. Use commercially available salivary substitutes or supplements (e.g., Salivart®, Salagen®, MoiStir®)

b)   Apply lip lubricant or mineral oil generously to patient's lips

  c) Keep patient's mouth and teeth clean

    i. Use soft-bristled toothbrushes or sponge-covered oral swabs with nonabrasive toothpaste to brush teeth

    ii. Tongue blade wrapped in gauze and moistened may be used as an alternative to a toothbrush

    iii. Keep dentures and bridges clean; do not insert if patient has mouth sores

    iv. Avoid alcohol-based mouthwashes and lemon glycerin swabs because of drying and unpleasant taste

    v. Frequently rinse mouth; mouth rinses using, for example, baking soda in water or saline rinses, chlorhexidine 0.2% (Peridex®)

    vi. Provide small chips of ice, frozen Gatorade™, or juice to refresh the patient

    vii. If the person is able to swallow, you can give him or her fluids in small amounts by syringe. However, carefully monitor for changes in the ability to swallow. Ensure that all family and healthcare team members are aware if a patient should NOT receive oral intake due to dysphagia

  d) Use topical (applied to the skin and mucous membranes) anesthetics (medications that numb an area, for example, lidocaine) for mouth sores

 2. Elimination management

  a) Use absorbent pads/adult diapers

  b) Apply moisture barrier to the skin

  c) Indwelling catheter for large amounts of urinary incontinence

  d) For fecal incontinence, assess for underlying causes, such as impaction, laxatives and tube feedings

 3. Skin integrity

  a) Watch for skin breakdown, especially in bony areas, such as shoulder blades, elbows, heels, back of head, over the ears and lower spine

  b) Prevent skin breakdown and discomfort through properly positioning the patient in bed and frequently turning the patient

  c) Be aware of the possible need to medicate the patient prior to turning her or him

  d) Anticipate the need for special pressure mattress for comfort and skin breakdown prevention before patient declines; this action may reduce the need for turning the patient in the final days or hours of life

  e) Use a turning sheet for lifting and turning the patient

f) If patient has skin breakdown

    i. Prevent further breakdown by carefully positioning the patient and frequently changing the patient's position

    ii. Observe the patient for pain or discomfort from the skin breakdown

    iii. Keep the area of the breakdown clean

    iv. Apply dressings as ordered

    v. Control wound odors by gently cleansing the area, applying and changing dressings appropriately, keeping room well ventilated, and using room deodorizers if necessary

V. Psychosocial and Spiritual Issues

A. Psychosocial Support for the Patient

1. Allow patients as much control over their environment and caregiving as possible

2. Maintain patient dignity

    a) Assume that the patient can hear all conversations; speak directly to the patient, even if she or he doesn't respond

    b) Adjust language; for example, speaking of "diapers" is not dignified

    c) Avoid speaking to others as if the patient were not present

3. Be aware of possible fears commonly experienced at the end of life, for example, fear of

    a) The unknown

    b) Being abandoned

    c) Being a burden to one's family or support system

4. Communication/support

    a) Listen carefully and address the patient's concerns

    b) Orient the patient frequently, even if patient is non-communicative

    c) Periodically assess the non-verbal patient's ability to communicate by other means, such as squeezing hands or blinking

B. Psychosocial Support for the Family

1. Listen carefully and address family concerns

2. Allow the family as much control over the environment as possible

3. When multiple family members are involved, be aware of who has the role of decision maker; and consult with that person regarding changes and decisions about the patient

4. Some families want to be present throughout the period when the patient is dying, whereas others are uncomfortable being near the person; respect individual preferences[1]

5.   Common family fears at time of the death of a loved one[2]

a)   Being alone with the patient

b)   Patient will have a painful death; having to watch patient suffer

c)   Being alone with patient when patient dies and fear of their own responses

d)   Not knowing when the patient is dead

e)   Causing the patient's death by giving medications (in home care setting)

C.   Grieving (also see Chapter XI)

1.   Grief

a)   Is an individual, emotional response to a loss

b)   Is a process that is not orderly or predictable

c)   Begins before the death occurs and continues after the death of the patient

2.   The grieving person never "gets over" a loss, but can heal and learn to live with a loss and live without the deceased

3.   Nursing actions

a)   Education and preparation

i.   Keep the family informed of the patient's status

ii.   Prepare the family for what to expect as the patient becomes closer to death

iii.   Provide information on grieving to help normalize the process

b)   Caregiving

i.   If the family wants to, encourage them to participate in caregiving

ii.   If family does not want to provide care or is emotionally or physically tired of caregiving, give them permission to take a break and allow others to provide patient care

iii.   By providing good care at the end of life, you help the patient to have a good death, which also eases grief for the family

c)   Grief coaching and resources

i.   Encourage families to communicate with the patient before death

ii.   Suggest that family members may wish to say good-bye when leaving the person, as death is unpredictable

iii.   Provide resources for available bereavement support

iv.   Provide spiritual support and referrals to clergy, as appropriate

D. Other Issues around Dying[4]

1. The "final rally"

   a) Days or hours before death, a non-verbal or comatose patient may suddenly awaken for a short time, be able to speak or even eat a meal

   b) Behavior is temporary, but may confuse family members as to the patient's status

2. Symbolic language

   a) Patient may talk about "preparing to go home," "going on a trip," "standing in line"

   b) Although the patient may seem confused, some healthcare workers see this as a normal process that they call "near-death awareness"

3. Vision-like experiences

   a) Person may experience seeing or speaking to persons who have already died; he or she may also see places not presently visible to others

   b) This normal process may reflect that the person is detaching from this life and is preparing for death

   c) Do not contradict, explain, belittle or argue about what the person claims to see or hear

4. Inability of the patient to let go

   a) Patient may perform repetitive and restless tasks

   b) May indicate that something is still unresolved or unfinished and preventing the letting go

   c) May need to talk with the team who can assist you and the family in identifying what may be happening and help the person find release from tension or fear

   d) As hard as it might be, the family may need to give the person permission to let go

5. Saying good-bye

   a) When the person is ready to die and the family is able to let go, saying good-bye is the final gift of love

   b) Saying good-bye achieves closure and may make the final release possible for the patient

   c) It may be helpful to encourage the family to hold or touch the patient and say the things that they want to say

      i. Message may be as simple (or as complicated) as saying, "I love you"

      ii. May include recounting favorite memories, places, and activities that were shared

      iii. May include saying "I'm sorry for whatever I've done to cause any tensions or difficulty"

      iv. Family members may also want to say "Thank you" and "I will miss you"

      v. Tears and crying are normal and natural part of saying good-bye, express loss and sadness and assure grieving people that there is no need to apologize or try to hide tears and sadness

6. Dying alone

    a) Family members may have a goal of being at the patient's bedside at the time of death and are upset it they are not present when the patient dies

    b) If this happens, gently explain this is not an uncommon occurrence

VI. Death

A. Signs that death is very near (hours or days) include

1. Changes in mentation

    a) Psychological and physical withdrawal

    b) Increased periods of sleeping

    c) Decreased consciousness

2. Lack of eyelash reflex indicates deep coma

3. Decreased and concentrated (dark) urinary output resulting from decreased blood circulation to the kidneys

4. Skin coolness; hands, arms, feet and legs become increasingly cool

5. Changes in skin color; paleness and sometimes presence of a bluish color resulting from decreased blood circulation

6. Incontinence; control of urine or bowels (or both) may be lost as the muscles in those areas begin to relax

7. Breathing pattern changes

    a) The person's regular breathing pattern may change and become irregular, e.g., shallow breaths with periods of no breathing for 5 to 30 seconds, up to a full minute, known as Cheyne-Stokes breathing

    b) Noisy respirations, death rattle

    c) Apnea, which is a period of no breathing

    d) Reinforce to family members that the above breathing patterns are an expected part of the dying process, and usually not distressful to patients

B. How will you know when death has occurred?

1. The signs of death include such things as

    a) No heartbeat

    b) Bowel and bladder incontinence

    c) No response

    d) Eyelids slightly open

    e) Pupils enlarged, do not respond to changes in light

    f)   Eyes fixed on a certain spot

    g)   No blinking

    h)   Jaw relaxed and mouth slightly open

2.   Talk with the family about what they should do if they are alone with the patient when the death occurs

    a)   The death of a hospice patient is expected and does not require an "emergency intervention." However, it often does require intense support for family at the bedside

    b)   Family or you should notify the team (hospice, on-call or unit)

    c)   The nurse will make the pronouncement and notify the physician and the funeral home

    d)   The body does not have to be moved until the family is ready

3.   Realize that even if the dying process is prolonged, you and the family may not be prepared for the actual moment

4.   Aftercare rituals and family support

    a)   Position the body in an appropriate way for family viewing

    b)   Help, if appropriate, with any cultural or religious rituals that the family desires

    c)   Encourage family to spend time with the body, saying good-byes

    d)   Ask if other family, friends, or clergy needs to come to view the body before post mortem care is performed

    e)   Reinforce teaching to family about what to expect

        i.   Rigor mortis (stiffening of the body after death) occurs 2 to 4 hours after death

        ii.   Air may escape lungs, especially when turning the body; assure family that this does not mean the patient is still alive

        iii.   Bowel and bladder incontinence commonly occur following death

5.   Post mortem care: care of the body after death

    a)   Handle the body with the same respect you would if the person were alive

    b)   Clean body and groom as appropriate

    c)   Ask if the family would like to participate in post mortem care; some family members find it comforting to perform this last act of care for a loved one; in some cultures and for some relationships (such as the death of a child), family participation in preparation of the body may be very important

    d)   Giving post mortem care provides a good opportunity for you to say your own "good-byes" to the patient

    e)   Prepare family members for the removal of the body from the room or home; this is often a difficult process to observe and families may wish to say good-byes and leave the area prior to the body being removed

VII. Professional Coping with Care of the Dying

A.   Recognize the importance of professional coping and self-care when working with the dying

B.   Reframe your view of dying, so that death is an expected part of your practice

C.   Acknowledge and explore your personal feelings about patients who die; find what works best for your coping

D.   Recognize your limits and ask for help when you need it

VIII. Conclusion

A.   Assist the patient to meet his or her own end-of-life goals (who, what, where)

B.   Enhance and individualize the environment

C.   Anticipate and monitor symptom management related to decline in status

D.   Anticipate psychosocial and spiritual care needs of patients and families

E.   Aid family grieving

F.   Recognize the importance of professional coping and self-care in working with the dying

CITED REFERENCES

1. American Association of Colleges of Nursing and the City of Hope National Medical Center. Module 8: Preparation and care for the time of death. *End-of-Life Nursing Education Consortium (ELNEC) project*, 2003: Funded through the Robert Wood Johnson Foundation.

2. Matzo ML. Peri-death Nursing Care. In: Matzo ML, Sherman DW. *Palliative Care Nursing: Quality Care to the End of Life*. New York, NY: Springer Publishing Company; 2001:487–517.

3. Ventafridda V, Ripamonte C, Shanotto A, De Conno F. Mouth care. In: Doyle D, Hanks GWC, MacDonald N, eds. *Oxford Textbook of Palliative Medicine*. 2nd ed. New York, NY: Oxford University Press; 1998:691–707.

4. Callahan M, Kelley P. *Final Gifts: Understanding the Special Awareness, Needs, & Communications of the Dying*. New York, NY: Bantam Books; 1992.

ADDITIONAL REFERENCES AND RESOURCES

Forbes MA, Rosdahl DR. The final journey of life. *Journal of Hospice and Palliative Nursing*. 2002:5(4):213–220.

Gauthier D. The meaning of healing near the end of life. *Journal of Hospice and Palliative Nursing*. 2002:4(4):220–227.

Kruse BG. The meaning of letting go: the lived experience for caregivers of persons at the end of life. *Journal of Hospice and Palliative Nursing*. 2002:6(4):215–222.

Ternestedt BM, Andershed B, Eriksson M, Johansson I. A good death: development of a nursing model of care. *Journal of Hospice and Palliative Nursing*. 2002:4(3):153–160.

Woods AB. The terror of the night: posttraumatic stress disorder at the end of life. *Journal of Hospice and Palliative Nursing*. 2002:5(4):196–204.

CHAPTER XIII

PERSONAL AND PROFESSIONAL DEVELOPMENT

Dena Jean Sutermaster, RN, MSN, CHPN®
Judy Lentz, RN, MSN, NHA

Adapted from: Poleto MA. Personal and Professional Development.
In: Ersek M, ed. *Core Curriculum for the Hospice and Palliative Nursing Assistant,*
Dubuque, IA: Kendall Hunt, 2003:115–123.

and

Rooney EC, Poleto M. Interdisciplinary Collaborative Practice in the Hospice and Palliative Care Setting.
In: Volker BG, Watson AC. eds. *Core Curriculum for the Generalist Hospice and Palliative Nurse.*
Dubuque, IA: Kendall/Hunt Publishing Company; 2002:15–28.

I.   **Introduction**[1]

    A.   Advances in the care of patients and family are always being developed

    B.   Licensed practical/vocational nurses must meet the basic education and training requirements for the licensed practical/vocational nurse job and also to remain current with information and procedures that are specific to the needs of the seriously ill and dying

    C.   Professional responsibilities go beyond maintaining one's competency and include other roles, such as advocating for patients, families, and colleagues; mentoring other licensed practical/vocational nurses and nursing assistants; and participating in activities aimed at improving care for seriously ill and dying patients and their families

II. Definitions

A. Professionalism[2]

1. As defined by National Board of Medical Examiners, professionalism is represented by the following characteristics

   a) Altruism

   b) Integrity

   c) Caring/compassion/communication

   d) Respect

   e) Responsibility/accountability

   f) Excellence/scholarship

   g) Leadership

2. Using this model for nurses practicing in end-of-life care, the professional nurse should demonstrate the following behaviors

   a) Altruism—put the patient/family first, continually advocate for the patient/family, be a team player promoting successful outcomes, participate in community activities that address end of life issues, and participate in local/national professional organizations

   b) Integrity—be truthful, do not withhold information, balance humility with authority, maintain professional autonomy

   c) Caring/compassion/communication—know when to listen, when to talk and when to seek additional information, break bad news with compassion; demonstrate compassion in every situation, show empathy

   d) Respect—respect patient/family rights requesting permission with any invasion of privacy, respect differences in culture, tradition, backgrounds, etc., maintain personal boundaries

   e) Responsibility/accountability—demonstrate reliability and accountability for responsibilities, be compliant with regulations and policies, be accountable for shortcomings, accept and provide constructive feedback, demonstrate ethical behaviors, control emotions with adversity

   f) Excellence/scholarship—be committed, conscientious, thorough, use good decision making skills, and continually seek to improve oneself scholastically

   g) Leadership—lead and mentor others, actively participate in activities within the specialty locally and nationally when possible, advocate for the profession, seek to grow professionally in every aspect, commit to the code of conduct, demonstrate competence and follow the standards of care and professional behavior as written for the specialty

B. Scope of Practice[1,3]

1. Activities the licensed practice/vocational nurse is legally permitted to perform as determined by their state board of nursing

2. Scope of hospice and palliative care licensed practical/vocational nurse is the distinct body of knowledge that directs the licensed practical/vocational nurse in providing hospice and palliative care

3. It is imperative that licensed practical/vocational nurses who work in hospice and palliative care accept professional practice accountability and make certain that their practice remain within the scope and professional practice standards

4. Licensed practical/vocational nurses practicing end-of-life care must have multidimensional skills and practice under the direction of a registered nurse

5. Licensed practical/vocational nurses can take on a variety of roles based on the needs of their patients and families

C. Hospice and palliative care standards of care[3]

1. Identifies the responsibilities for which hospice and palliative care licensed practical/vocational nurse is accountable

2. Describe a competent level of licensed practical/vocational nursing care as demonstrated by the nursing process

D. Competencies for the hospice and palliative care licensed practical/vocational nurse[4]

1. In the *Professional Competencies for the Hospice and Palliative Licensed Practical/Vocational Nurse* professionalism is defined as one who "demonstrates knowledge, attitudes, behaviors and skills that are consistent with the scope of practice for hospice and palliative licensed practical/vocational nursing."[4, p.3] The core competencies for professionalism in hospice and palliative nursing as defined by the Hospice and Palliative Nurses Association are

   a) Recognizes that influence of personal spiritual and cultural values on perceptions regarding dying and death and their impact on the quality of hospice and palliative care

   b) Demonstrates caring behavior and interpersonal connectiveness while maintaining personal and professional boundaries

   c) Demonstrates professional accountability to patients, families, colleagues and institutions

   d) Engages in nursing activities that are appropriate to personal education, experience and scope of practice

   e) Supports the advancement of hospice/palliative nursing through membership in HPNA and other professional organizations and participation in hospice and palliative education and community activities

   f) Participates in ongoing educational activities and certification to promote professional development

g)   Seeks constructive feedback regarding ones' own professional practice through participation on performance evaluation, peer review and interactions with colleagues

h)   Maintains physical, social, emotional and spiritual care of self

i)   Delegates and supervises care responsibilities within the individual's scope of practice and/or other regulatory parameters

E.   Professional Growth and Development

1.   Maintain professional boundaries

a)   Understand team roles and work within them maintaining flexibility and willingness to blend roles as needed

b)   Set boundaries/limits for self and others in patient/family relationships

c)   Respond appropriately to those who overstep these boundaries

d)   Foster independence in patients and families

2.   Provide self care through stress management

a)   Assess self care strategies

b)   Acknowledge potential stress/presence of stress

c)   Recognize ways to relieve stress

d)   Practice spiritual self care

e)   Actively participate in stress management

f)   Seek assistance of others when indicated

g)   Maintain a balanced life

h)   Develop and maintain a strong support system

i)   Stay involved with the team dynamics for support and understanding

3.   Participate in peer review and development

a)   Seek ways to precept, educate and mentor others

b)   Support and guide coworkers in clinical practice growth and development

c)   Accept the support of others

d)   Assist in developing mentoring programs

4.   Commit to self growth

a)   Commit to continuing education through journals, conferences, educational opportunities

b)   Commit to membership in professional specialty organizations and participate in the activities provided locally, regionally and nationally

c)   Participate and support research efforts to establish evidence based outcomes incorporating these outcomes into practice

F. Mentor[1,5]

1. Can be in a formal relationship such as orientation or informally as assistant

2. Individual having advanced knowledge and experience in an area of work who shares this knowledge with a newer team member

3. Mentors may not necessarily work side-by-side with the newer coworker, but are available to listen, support, and guide the newer co-worker to become more familiar with the job and agency processes

G. Networking[1,5]

1. Communication with other hospice and palliative care team members

2. Allows for opportunity to share information about hospice and palliative care in general and particular cases with colleagues

3. May happen in a variety of settings, e.g., at lunch or in the report room, also at conferences and meetings

4. Connections made between people of similar backgrounds

5. Provides opportunities to discuss similar problems and solutions; decreases feelings of isolation

6. On-line through Special Interest Group listservs and HPNA Forum

H. Certification[1,5]

1. Professional recognition of hospice and palliative nursing knowledge through the successfully completing an examination

2. Process through which a professional group validates an individual's qualifications and knowledge in the specialized area of practice

3. The National Board for Certification of Hospice and Palliative Nurses (NBCHPN®) began certifying LP/VNs in September 2004. LP/VNs who are certified use the credential of CHPLN

4. Hospice and palliative certification is separate from licensure and is voluntary. It is not required by law for practice

5. Recertification every four years maintains the credibility of this knowledge

I. Advocacy[1,5]

1. Process and act of representing the wishes, values, or concerns of another individual who may be less able to do so

2. Advocates must have knowledge of the person's wishes, etc. and be assertive in stating those wishes to others

J. Collaboration[1]

1. Working together with other individuals in a positive and effective manner where the combination of the knowledge and gifts of each individual in the group results in better outcomes for the patient and family

2. Requires open communication, mutual respect, and similar goals or mission

K. Quality improvement[6]

1. A commitment and a systemic approach to improve every process in every part of an organization: goal is to exceed customer's (usually patient and family) expectations of care

2. Is a process to identify and solve problems with a goal to improve care and patient outcomes

3. Example of QI (Quality Improvement) Model: the Plan-Do-Check-Act (PDCA) Cycle: Steps[1,6-8]

   a) Plan: identify a problem (e.g., families reluctance to give opioid pain medications); design an approach to solve problems or improve outcomes (e.g., work with team to teach staff to ask families why they are reluctant to give pain medication and to talk to the families about how pain medications work; assist team to develop a teaching sheet on opioid pain medications)

   b) Do: institute the change and collect information about the effect of the changes on practice and outcomes (e.g., work with team to determine use of opioid pain medications and levels of pain following changes)

   c) Check: analyze the results (e.g., with team compare the use of opioid pain medication and pain levels before and after the change; did they decease, increase or stay the same?)

   d) Act: if the changes resulted in better outcomes, then plan ways to maintain the positive gains; if outcomes didn't change or get worse, develop different ways to approach the problem and test these approaches (e.g., if staff education and teaching sheets didn't work, the agency could develop a formal procedure for discussing opioid pain medication with families)

4. Research[1]

   a) A systematic study or examination of a problem or question

   b) Similar to QI, but usually more detailed

   c) Research can take many forms: interviews, surveys, physical and chemical measures (e.g., blood pressure, pain, laboratory values)

   d) Reported in professional journals and presentations

III. Professional Expectations and Development

A. Achieving and Maintaining Competency: Education and Training[1]

1. Licensed practical/vocational nurses must graduate from an education program approved by their state board of nursing

2. Licensed practical/vocational nurses must pass the NCLEX-PN®

3. Licensed practical/vocational nurses should complete specific in-services and competency evaluation for the licensed practical/vocational nurse in hospice and palliative care

4. Licensed practical/vocational nurses should participate in optional learning experiences to maintain expertise

   a) Read professional journals, newsletters and websites

   b) View educational videotapes

   c) Attend classes on topics related to hospice and palliative care

5. Maintain personal continuing education plan to update knowledge

   a) Track attendance at conferences and meetings

   b) List educational opportunities by title and presenter

   c) Retain copies of handouts and number of hours attended

6. Licensed practical/vocational nurses are encouraged to continue their formal education in nursing and/or other professional disciplines. Programs in further education in nursing can include

   a) Registered nursing (RN)—after attending either a diploma program, associate degree program or bachelor's program, nurses must successfully complete the NCLEX-RN® to practice as an RN

      i. Diploma programs—affiliated with a hospital and are around 24 months in length

      ii. Associate Degree programs (ADN)—affiliated with community/junior colleges and are 2 years in length

      iii. Bachelor of Science in Nursing (BSN)—affiliated with colleges and universities and are 4 years in length

      iv. RN to BSN—a program offered by some colleges and universities to facilitate the achievement of a bachelor's degree for RNs

   b) Masters (MSN, MN)

      i. Offered by numerous colleges and universities in many specialties to prepare nurses with BSNs to practice in advanced nursing roles. Length is usually at least 2 years, but depends on field of study. Examples can include

         (a) Clinical nurse specialist—manages patient care at an advanced practice level

         (b) Nurse practitioner—delivers advanced practice nursing care independently

         (c) Education—preparation for teaching nurses in schools of nursing or staff development

    c)   Doctorate (PhD)—offered by universities to prepare nurses with an MSN or MN to do research

B.   Mentoring[1,5]

1.   Licensed practical/vocational nurses should mentor other licensed practical/vocational nurses and nursing assistants in work place to share experiences and provide support and friendship

2.   Licensed practical/vocational nurses should help and participate in in-services, orientation and other programs

3.   Mentor student nurses, social worker and chaplain interns, medical students and others

4.   Precept new staff and provide guidance and support

5.   Assist in the development and evaluation of preceptor/mentor programs

C.   Networking and professional relationships[1,5]

1.   Licensed practical/vocational nurses should participate in membership organizations that promote quality nursing care, e.g., Hospice and Palliative Nurses Association

2.   Licensed practical/vocational nurses should volunteer for committees at work and for professional organizations

3.   Network with peers to share information and promote connectedness within the professional

D.   Certification[1]

1.   Certification assists in meeting professional expectations by providing educational, networking, mentoring and advocacy opportunities

2.   Involves meeting eligibility requirements and passing a standardized test that reflects a national standard of knowledge needed to provide quality hospice and palliative licensed practical/vocational nursing care

E.   Advocacy[1]

1.   Licensed practical/vocational nurses should listen carefully to learn patients' and families' goals and values

2.   Licensed practical/vocational nurses should learn assertive communication skills to share patients' and families goals with other team members

3.   Licensed practical/vocational nurses should remind team members and community about the importance of the licensed practical/vocational nurse in hospice and palliative care as a team member

4.   Licensed practical/vocational nurses should support fellow licensed practical/vocational nurses when they have good ideas about improving care of the seriously ill and dying

5.   Licensed practical/vocational nurses should volunteer/join local or regional groups that focus on quality care of the seriously ill and dying

F.   Quality Improvement (QI)[1]

    1.   Licensed practical/vocational nurses should participate in QI activities at work; volunteer for the QI committee

        a)   Provide ideas and feedback on agency processes and practices that could be improved to serve the patient and family

        b)   Report problems or issues that have (or potentially have) a negative or harmful impact on patient, families and staff

G.   Research[1,5]

    1.   Licensed practical/vocational nurses should volunteer to gather data and information as directed by the research team

    2.   Licensed practical/vocational nurses should assist in using research findings in practice

    3.   Critical steps in research

        a)   Develop an idea

        b)   Define the problem/issue/question

        c)   Collect background information

        d)   Develop a written plan

        e)   State objectives or hypothesis

        f)   Determine research design

        g)   Collect data

        h)   Analyze data

        i)   Draw conclusions

        j)   Apply findings to clinical practice as appropriate

        k)   Disseminate findings to colleagues

H.   Read medical and nursing journals to remain current in knowledge of treatment options and end-of-life care[5]

    1.   Peer reviewed—more formal articles with extensive literature reviews that are reviewed by content experts for accurateness before being published

        a)   Research articles—peer reviewed article that is based on an individual or groups research study

    2.   Non-peer reviewed—less formal articles based on personal opinion or experiences

I.   Participate in professional nursing organization activities[5]

    1.   Hospice and Palliative Nurses Association

        a)   National

        b)   Chapters

2. State organizations

3. LP/VN organizations include

   a) National Association of Practical Nursing Education and Service, Inc.

   b) National Federation of Licensed Practical Nurses, Inc.

4. Attend state and national conferences

5. Obtain certification in specialty areas of practice, i.e., hospice and palliative nursing

J.   Participate in peer review

1. Participate in peer review process according to agency's policies

K.   Maintain professional boundaries between patients/family and staff[5]

1. Understand team members roles

2. Maintaining boundaries minimizes conflict

3. Work within defined role limits as appropriate, but be flexible, able and willing to blend roles when necessary

4. Each team member should be aware of need to set limits/boundaries for self and others when interacting with patients and families

5. Foster independence of patients and families; empower them to maintain maximum control of their lives

IV.   Addressing Professional Stresses

A.   Sources of stress for professional caregivers at the end of life[1]

1. Your own grief

2. Personal comfort level with dying

3. Feeling of helplessness

4. Sense that others don't care as much as you do

5. Lack of time to provide the care that you want to

6. Accept that stress exists and will be experienced by everyone who works with the dying and their families

7. Acknowledge that people often do not recognize stress in themselves

B.   Manifestations of stress[1]

   1.   Physical distress and fatigue

   2.   Feeling irritable a lot of the time

   3.   Emotional withdrawal from persons you are caring for

   4.   Trouble with personal relationships

   5.   Starting to feel like you are the only one who can give good care

C.   Interventions to prevent and decrease job-related stress[1,5]

   1.   Recognize that everyone on the team needs each other; no one is giving care alone

   2.   Start or maintain physical exercise program

   3.   Take care of your own emotional and spiritual needs

   4.   Find people whom you feel comfortable talking to about feelings

   5.   Recognize that you can't be or do everything for everyone; remember that even "Superman" is Clark Kent most of the time!

   6.   Be aware that clinical competency helps to reduce stress—take advantage of educational opportunities

   7.   Increase knowledge regarding end-of-life care, bereavement support and public policy affecting end-of-life care

   8.   Develop and maintain strong personal support systems

   9.   Maintain a balance in interactions with patients and families. Self-awareness is important in maintenance of appropriate boundaries

  10.   Secure a sense of closure after patients' deaths

  11.   Get adequate rest, eat a proper diet and participate in regular physical exercise

  12.   Remain involved with the team for mutual support and a feeling of belonging

D.   Advocate for the profession[5]

   1.   Keep informed about the state and federal policies that impact end-of-life care

   2.   Know and support various professional organizations' position statements on end-of-life care; maintain open dialogue on this topic

   3.   Educate policy makers, legislators about the needs of families experiencing end-of-life care

CITED REFERENCES

1.   Poleto MA. Personal and professional development. In: Ersek M. ed. *Core Curriculum for the Hospice and Palliative Nursing Assistant.* Dubuque, IA: Kendall/Hunt Publishing Company; 2003:115–123.

2.   National Board of Medical Examiners. The Behaviors of Professionalism. Available at http://ci.nbme.org/professionalism/behaviors.asp. Accessed May 17, 2004.

3.   Dahlin C, Lentz J, Sutermaster DJ. *Statement of the Scope and Standards of Hospice and Palliative Licensed Practical/Vocational Nursing Practice.* Dubuque, IA: Kendall/Hunt Publishing Company; 2004.

4.   Dahlin C, Lentz J, Sutermaster DJ. *Professional Competencies for the Hospice and Palliative Licensed Practical/Vocational Nurse.* Dubuque, IA: Kendall/Hunt Publishing Company; 2004.

5.   Rooney EC, Poleto M. Interdisciplinary Collaborative Practice in the Hospice and Palliative Care Setting. In: Volker BG, Watson AC. eds. *Core Curriculum for the Generalist Hospice and Palliative Nurse.* Dubuque, IA: Kendall/Hunt Publishing Company; 2002:15–28.

6.   Bookbinder M. Improving the quality of care across all settings. In: Ferrell BR, Coyle N. *Textbook of Palliative Nursing.* New York, NY: Oxford University Press; 2001:503–530.

7.   Deming WE. *Out of the Crisis.* Cambridge, MA: Massachusetts Institute of Technology Center for Advanced Engineering Study; 1986.

8.   Nelson EC, Batalden PB, Ryer JC. eds. *Joint Commission Clinical Improvement Action Guide.* Oakbrook Terrace, IL: The Joint Accreditation of Healthcare Organizations; 1998.

ADDITIONAL REFERENCES AND RESOURCES

Gaydos H, Lee B. The living end: life journeys of hospice nurses. *Journal of Hospice and Palliative Nursing.* 2002:17–26.

Quaglietti S, Blum L, Ellis V. The role of the adult nurse practitioner in palliative care. *Journal of Hospice and Palliative Nursing.* 2002:6(4):209–214.

Tyree TL, Long CO, Greenberg EA. Nurse practitioners and end-of-life care: beliefs, practices and perceptions. *Journal of Hospice and Palliative Nursing.* 2002:7(1):45–51.

WEBSITE/INTERNET RESOURCES[1]

Agency for Healthcare Research and Quality	http://www.ahcpr.gov/
Aging with Dignity	http://www.agingwithdignity.org
American Academy of Hospice and Palliative Medicine	http://www.aahpm.org
American Academy of Pain Medicine	http://www.painmed.org
American Alliance of Cancer Pain Initiatives	http://www.aacpi.org/resource.html
American Association for Therapeutic Humor	http://www.aath.org
American Board of Internal Medicine Care for the Dying, Physician Narratives—	http://www.abim.org/pubs/narr001.htm
American Cancer Society	http://www.cancer.org
American Chronic Pain Association	http://www.theacpa.org/
American Council for Headache Education	http://www.achenet.org
The American Geriatrics Society	http://www.americangeriatrics.org
American Holistic Nurses Association	http://www.ahna.org
American Massage Therapy Association	http://www.amtamassage.org
American Medical Association	http://www.ama-assn.org.
American Medical Association Education of Physicians on End of Life Care (EPEC)	http://www.ama-assn.org/ama/pub/category/2719.html
American Music Therapy Association	http://www.namt.com
American Pain Foundation	http://www.painfoundation.org
American Pain Society	http://www.ampainsoc.org
American Society of Anesthesiologists	http://www.asahq.org

American Society for Bioethics and Humanities	http://www.asbh.org
American Society of Clinical Oncology (ASCO)	http://www.asco.org
American Society of Law, Medicine and Ethics	http://www.aslme.org
American Society of Pain Management Nurses	http://www.aspmn.org
Approaching Death: Improving Care at the End of Life	http://www.nap.edu/readingroom/books/approaching/
Arthritis Foundation	http://www.arthritis.org
Association of Cancer Online Resources, Inc.	http://www.acor.org
Association for Death Education and Counseling (ADEC)	http://www.adec.org
Association of Nurses in AIDS Care	http://www.anacnet.org
Association of Oncology Social Work (AOSW)	http://www.aosw.org
Association of Pediatric Oncology Nurses (APON)	http://www.apon.org
Before I Die: Medical Care and Personal Choices	http://www.wnet.org/archive/bid
Cancer Care®	http://www.cancercare.org
CancerLink	http://www.personal.u-et.com/~njh/cancer.html
National Cancer Institute Cancer Topics	http://www.cancer.gov/cancerinformation
Candlelighters Childhood Cancer Foundation	http://www.candlelighters.org
Caregiver Network Inc.	http://www.caregiver.on.ca/index.html
Catholic Health Association of the United States	http://www.chausa.org
Center to Improve Care of the Dying	http://www.gwu.edu/~cicd
Children's Hospice International	http://www.chionline.org
Choices	http://www.choices.org
City of Hope Pain/Palliative Care Resource Center	http://prc.coh.org
The Compassionate Friends Inc.	http://www.compassionatefriends.org/
U. S. Department of Health and Human Services, Healthfinder®	http://www.healthfinder.gov
Dying Well	http://www.dyingwell.org
Education for Physicians on End of Life Care Project (EPEC)	http://www.epec.net
The End of Life: Exploring Death in America	http://www.npr.org/programs/death/
End of Life / Palliative Education Resource Center (EPERC)	http://www.eperc.mcw.edu
FACCT—Foundation for Accountability	http://www.facct.org
Family Caregiver Alliance®	http://www.caregiver.org
Fibromyalgia Network	http://www.fmnetnews.com

Geronurse Online	http://www.geronurseonline.org
Growth House, Inc.	http://www.growthhouse.org
Hospice Association of America	http://www.hospice-america.org
Hospice and Palliative Nurses Association	http://www.hpna.org
Hospice Foundation of America (HFA)	http://www.hospicefoundation.org
Hospice Cares Pharmacy	http://www.hospice-cares.com
Institute for Healthcare Improvement	http://www.ihi.org
International Association for the Study of Pain®	http://www.iasp-pain.org/
Leukemia & Lymphoma Society®	http://www.leukemia.org
Make a Wish Foundation®	http://www.wish.org
Medical College of Wisconsin: Center for the Study of Bioethics	http://www.mcw.edu/bioethics/
Medical College of Wisconsin: Palliative Care Center	http://www.mcw.edu/pallmed/
Memorial Sloan-Kettering Cancer Center	http://www.mskcc.org
The Nathan Cummings Foundation	http://www.ncf.org/index.html
National Association for Home Care and Hospice (NAHC)	http://www.nahc.org/
The National Center for Health Statistics	http://www.cdc.gov/nchs/about.htm
National Conference of State Legislatures	http://www.ncsl.org/programs/pubs/endoflife.htm
National Family Caregivers Association	http://www.nfcacares.org/
National Hospice and Palliative Care Organization	http://www.nhpco.org
The National Institute on Aging	http://www.nih.gov/nia/
National Prison Hospice Association	http://www.npha.org
The Neuropathy Association	http://www.neuropathy.org
New York State Partnership for Long-Term Care	http://www.nyspltc.org/about/index.html#3
Not Dead Yet	http://www.notdeadyet.org/
On Our Own Terms	http://www.thirteen.org/onourownterms
OncoLink	http://www.oncolink.com
Open Society Institute	http://www.soros.org
Oregon Health Sciences University Center for Ethics in Health Care	http://www.ohsu.edu/ethics/
Oncology Nursing Society	http://www.ons.org
PainLink	http://www.edc.org/PainLink
Pain Net, Inc.	http://www.painnet.com
Partners Against Pain®	http://www.partnersagainstpain.com

Patient Education Institute	http://www.patient-education.com
Pediatric Pain	http://is.dal.ca/~pedpain/prohp.html
Pediatric Pain Education for Patients & Families	http://pedspain.nursing.uiowa.edu
Reflex Sympathetic Dystrophy Association of California	http://www.rsdsa-ca.org/
Regional Palliative Care Program in Edmunton Alberta	http://www.palliative.org
The Robert Wood Johnson Foundation	http://www.rwjf.org
Sickle Cell Disease Association of American, Inc.	http://www.sicklecelldisease.org
Southern California Cancer Pain Initiative (SCCPI)	http://sccpi.coh.org
Supportive Care of the Dying	http://www.careofdying.org
TMJ Association, Ltd.	http://www.tmj.org
TALARIA: The Hypermedia Assistant for Cancer Pain Management	http://www.stat.washington.edu/TALARIA/talariahome.html
Telemedicine Information Exchange	http://tie.telemed.org
Today's Caregiver Magazine	http://www.caregiver.com/
United Hospital Fund of New York	http://www.uhfnyc.org
University of Wisconsin Pain & Policy Studies Group	http://www.medsch.wisc.edu/painpolicy/
VistaCare	http://www.vista-care.com
Task Force on Life & the Law: When Death is Sought	http://www.health.state.ny.us/nysdoh/provider/death.htm
Wisconsin Pain Initiative	http://www.aacpi.wisc.edu/wcpi
World Health Organization	http://www.who.int/en

APPENDIX 2

COMMONLY USED MEDICATIONS
Trade and Generic Names

ALZHEIMER'S DRUGS

Aricept® . . . . donepezil
Cognex® . . . . tacrine
Exelon® . . . . rivastigmine
Namenda® . . . . memantine
Reminyl® . . . . galantamine

ANALGESICS

Actiq® . . . . fentanyl citrate
Avinza®/Kadian®/MS Contin®/
 Oramorph® SR/Roxanol® . . . . morphine sulfate
Dilaudid®/Palladone™ . . . . hydromorphone
Dolophine® . . . . methadone
Duragesic® . . . . fentanyl transdermal system
Empirin w/Codeine®/Tylenol w/Codeine® . . . . . aspirin/codeine
Fiorinal® . . . . aspirin/caffeine/butalbital
Lidoderm HCL Topical® . . . . lidocaine
Levo-Dromoran® . . . . levorphanol
Oxycontin®/OxyFAST® . . . . oxycodone
Percocet®/Roxicet® . . . . oxycodone/acetaminophen
Percodan® . . . . oxycodone/aspirin
Tylenol® . . . . acetaminophen
Ultram® . . . . tramadol
Vicodin®/Lorcet® . . . . hydrocodone/acetaminophen

ANTACIDS/ANTIFLATULANTS/DIGESTANTS

Basaljel® . . . . aluminum carbonate gel
Carafate® . . . . sucralfate
Gelusil® . . . . aluminum hydroxide/magnesium hydroxide/simethicone
Maalox® . . . . magnesium hydroxide/aluminum hydroxide
Mylanta® . . . . magnesium hydroxide/aluminum hydroxide/simethicone
Mylicon® . . . . simethicone
Pancrease®/Viokase® . . . . pancrelipase

---

* "Tall Man" lettering as suggested by the FDA to differentiate look-alike medication names.

ANTIANGINAL

Calan®/Isoptin®	verapamil
Isordil®	isosorbide dinitrate
Cardizem®	diltiazem
Persantine®	dipyridamole
Procardia®	NIFEdipine*

ANTIBIOTICS

Ancef®	cefazolin
Augmentin®	amoxicillin
Bactrim®	trimethoprim/sulfamethoxazole
Biaxin®	clarithromycin
Ceclor®	cefaclor
Cefobid®	cefoperazone
Ceftin®	cefuroxime
Claforan®	cefotaxime
Cleocin®	clindamycin
Fortaz®	ceftazidime
Garamycin®	gentamicin
Rocephin®	ceftriaxone
Timentin®	ticarcillin/clavulanate
Unasyn®	ampicillin/sulbactam
Zithromax®	azithromycin
Zosyn®	piperacillin/tazobactam

ANTICOAGULANTS

Coumadin®	warfarin
Lovenox®	enoxaparin

ANTICONVULSANTS

Depacon®	valproate
Depakote®	valproic acid
Dilantin®	phenytoin
Keppra®	levetiracetam
Klonopin®	clonazepam
Lamictal®	lamotrigine
Mysoline®	primidone
Neurontin®	gabapentin
Tegretol®	carbamazepine
Topamax®	topiramate
Zonegran®	zonisamide

ANTIDEPRESSANTS

Adepin®/Sinequan®	doxepin
Celexa®	citalopram
Cymbalta®	duloxetine
Desyrel®	trazodone
Effexor®	venlafaxine
Elavil®/Endep®	amitriptyline
Lexapro®	escitalopram
Luvox®	fluvoxamine

Norpramin® .... desipramine
Pamelor® .... nortriptyline
Paxil® .... paroxetine
Prozac® .... fluoxetine
Remeron® .... mirtazapine
Serzone® .... nefazodone
Surmontil® .... trimipramine
Tofranil® .... imipramine
Tofranil® PM .... imipramine pamoate
Vivactil® .... protriptylin
Wellbutrin® .... buPROPion*
Zoloft® .... sertraline

ANTIDIABETICS
Amary® .... glimepiride
Diabinese® .... chlorproPAMIDE*
Glucotrol®/Glucotrol® .... glipiZIDE*
Glynase®/Micronase® .... glyBURIDE*
Orinase® .... TOLBUTamide*
Prandin® .... repaglinide
Starlix® .... nateglinide
Tolinase® .... TOLAZamide*

ANTIDIARRHEAL
Donnagel®/Kaopectate® .... kaolin/pectin
Imodium® .... loperamide
Lomotil® .... diphenoxylate/atropine
Pepto-Bismol® .... bismuth subsalicylate
Paregoric® .... camphorated opium tincture
Sandostatin® .... octreotide

ANTIFUNGAL
Diflucan® .... fluconazole
Flagyl® .... metronidazole
Monistat® .... miconazole nitrate
Mycelex®/Lotrimin® .... clotrimazole
Nizoral® .... ketoconazole
Mycostatin® .... nystatin
Sporanox® .... itraconazole

ANTIGOUT
Benemid® .... probenecid
Zyloprim®/Lopurin® .... allopurinol

ANTIHYPERTENSIVES
Capoten® .... captopril
Corgard® .... nadolol
Inderal® .... propranolol
Lopressor® .... metoprolol
Prinivil®/Zestril® .... lisinopril
Tenormin® .... atenolol

Trandate® . . . . labetalol
Vasotec® . . . . enalapril

ANTIHYSTAMINES
Allegra® . . . . fexofenadine
Atarax® . . . . hydrOXYzine*
Benadryl® . . . . diphenhydrAMINE*
Chlor-Trimeton® . . . . chlorpheniramine
Clarinex® . . . . desloratadine
Claritin®/Alavert® . . . . loratadine
Tavist® . . . . clemastine
Zyrtec® . . . . cetirizine

ANTINAUSEA/ANTIEMETIC/PROMOTILITY
Aloxi® . . . . palonosetron
Antivert® . . . . meclizine
Anzemet® . . . . dolasetron
Compazine® . . . . prochlorperazine
Dramamine® . . . . dimenhyDRINATE*
Emend® . . . . aprepitant
Haldol® . . . . haloperidol
Kytril® . . . . granisetron
Phenergan® . . . . promethazine
Reglan® . . . . metoclopramide
Thorazine® . . . . chlorproMAZINE*
Tigan® . . . . trimethobenzamide
Torecan® . . . . thiethylperazine
Trilafon® . . . . perphenazine
Zofran® . . . . ondansetron

ANTIPARKINSON AGENTS
Apokyn® . . . . apomorphine
Artane® . . . . trihexyphenidyl
Cogentin® . . . . benztropine
Mirapex® . . . . pramipexole
Parlodel® . . . . bromocriptine
Permax® . . . . pergolide
Sinemet® . . . . carbidopa/levodopa
Stalevo® . . . . carbidopa/levodopa/entacapone
Symmetrel® . . . . amantadine

ANTIPRURITICS
Caladryl® . . . . calamine/diphenhydrAMINE*

ANTIPSYCHOTICS
Clozaril® . . . . clozapine
Haldol® . . . . haloperidol
Loxitane® . . . . loxapine
Mellaril® . . . . thioridazine
Moban® . . . . molindone
Navane® . . . . thiothixene

Prolixin® . . . . fluphenazine
Risperdal® . . . . risperidone
Seroquel® . . . . quetiapine
Stelazine® . . . . trifluoperazine
Thorazine® . . . . chlorproMAZINE*
Trilafon® . . . . perphenazine
Zyprexa® . . . . olanzapine

ANTISECRETORY/ANTICHOLINERGIC
Levsin® . . . . hyoscyamine
Transderm-Scop® . . . . scopolamine

ANTIVIRAL
Famvir® . . . . famciclovir
Valtrex® . . . . valacyclovir
Zovirax® . . . . acyclovir

ANXIOLYTIC/ANTIDEPRESSANT
Etrafon®/Triavil® . . . . perphenazine/amitriptyline

ANXIOLYTIC/SEDATIVE
Ambien® . . . . zolpidem
Ativan® . . . . lorazepam
Zydis®/Zyprexa® . . . . olanzapine
BuSpar® . . . . busPIRone
Dalmane® . . . . flurazepam
Halcion® . . . . triazolam
Klonopin® . . . . clonazepam
Librium® . . . . chlordiazepoxide
Nembutal® . . . . pentobarbital
Placidyl® . . . . ethchlorvynol
Restoril® . . . . temazepam
Seconal® . . . . secobarbital
Serax® . . . . oxazepam
Sonata® . . . . zaleplon
Tranxene® . . . . clorazepate
Valium® . . . . diazepam
Versed® . . . . midazolam

APPETITE STIMULANT
Megace® . . . . megestrol

BISPHOSPHONATES
Aredia® . . . . pamidronate
Zometa® . . . . zoledronic acid

CARDIAC GLYCOSIDES
Lanoxin® . . . . digoxin

H₂ BLOCKERS/PROTON PUMP INHIBITORS

Nexium® . . . . esomeprazole
Pepcid® . . . . famotidine
Prevacid® . . . . lansoprazole
Prilosec® . . . . omeprazole
Protonix® . . . . pantoprazole
Tagamet® . . . . cimetidine
Zantac® . . . . ranitidine

LAXATIVES

Benefiber® . . . . soluble fiber
CitroMag® . . . . magnesium citrate
Citrucel® . . . . methylcellulose
Chronulac® . . . . lactulose
Colace®/Surfak®/Regutol® . . . . docusate sodium
Dulcolax® . . . . bisacodyl
Fiberall®/FiberCon® . . . . calcium polycarbophil
Fleet Enema® . . . . sodium biphosphate/phosphate
Metamucil® . . . . psyllium
MiraLax™ . . . . polyethylene glycol
Phillips' Milk of Magnesia® . . . . magnesium hydroxide
Senokot® . . . . senna

MUSCLE RELAXANTS

Flexeril® . . . . cyclobenzaprine
Lioresal® . . . . baclofen
Norflex® . . . . orphenadrine
Robaxin® . . . . methocarbamol
Soma® . . . . carisprodol
Quinamm® . . . . quinine sulfate
Valium, Valrelease® . . . . diazepam

NSAIDs

Aleve®/Anaprox®/Naprosyn® . . . . naproxen sodium
Celebrex® . . . . celecoxib
Indocin® . . . . indomethacin
Motrin® . . . . ibuprofen
Trilisate® . . . . choline magnesium trisalicylate

PSYCHOSTIMULANTS

Dexedrine® . . . . dextroamphetamine
Provigil® . . . . modafinil
Ritalin® . . . . methylphenidate

STEROIDS

Decadron® . . . . dexamethasone
Deltasone® . . . . predniSONE*
Orapred®/Prelone® . . . . prednisoLONE*
Medrol®/Solu-Medrol® . . . . methylPRED-NISolone*
Solu-Cortef® . . . . hydrocortisone

References

Skidmore-Roth L. *2005 Mosby's Nursing Drug Reference.* St. Louis, MO, Inc.; 2005.

APPENDIX 3

STANDARDS OF HOSPICE AND PALLIATIVE CARE LICENSED PRACTICAL/VOCATIONAL NURSING

Standards of Care

Standard I: Data Gathering
The hospice and palliative care licensed practical/vocational nurse collects patient and family data.

Standard II: Outcome Identification
The hospice and palliative care licensed practical/vocational nurse identifies expected outcomes relevant to the individual and family and with the interdisciplinary/healthcare team, when appropriate.

Standard III: Planning
The hospice and palliative care licensed practical/vocational nurse assists with developing a plan of care that is negotiated among the individual, family, and interdisciplinary/healthcare team that includes interventions and treatments to attain expected outcomes.

Standard IV: Implementation
The hospice and palliative care licensed practical/vocational nurse implements the interventions identified in the plan of care.

Standard V: Evaluation
The hospice and palliative care licensed practical/vocational nurse evaluates the individuals' and families' progress in attaining expected outcomes.

Standards of Professional Performance

Standard I: Quality of Care
The hospice and palliative care licensed practical/vocational nurse systematically evaluates the quality and effectiveness of care.

Standard II: Performance Appraisal
The hospice and palliative care licensed practical/vocational nurse evaluates one's own practice in relation to professional practice standards and relevant standards and regulations.

Standard III: Education
The hospice and palliative care licensed practical/vocational nurse acquires and maintains current knowledge and competency in hospice and palliative care nursing.

Standard IV: Collegiality
The hospice and palliative licensed practical/vocational nurse interacts and contributes to the professional development of peers and other healthcare providers as colleagues.

Standard V: Ethics
The hospice and palliative care licensed practical/vocational nurse makes decisions and acts on behalf of patient and family in an ethical manner.

Standard VI: Collaboration
The hospice and palliative care licensed practical/vocational nurse collaborates with patient and family, members of the interdisciplinary/healthcare team and other healthcare providers in providing patient and family care.

Standard VII: Resource Utilization
The hospice and palliative care licensed practical/vocational nurse considers factors related to safety, effectiveness, and cost in planning and delivering patient and family care.